Children
Who
Grieve

CHILDREN WHO GRIEVE

Roberta Beckmann

LP Learning Publications, Inc.
MONTREAL   HOLMES BEACH, FL

ISBN 1-55691-050-9

Learning Publications, Inc.
5351 Gulf Drive
P.O. Box 1338
Holmes Beach, FL 34218-1338

Printing: 10 9 8 7   Year: 10 9 8 7

Printed in the United States of America.

This Book is Lovingly

Dedicated to:

My father, Lester Albin
My mother, Velda Albin
My brother, Lloyd Albin

for whom I loved
and
for whom I grieved when they died.

My sons, Jon Paul and Jason
who have taught me about children
and about loving more deeply.

Table of Contents

PREFACE

As with adults, grief is difficult for children. They need adults to love them, to understand what they are going through, to encourage them, to listen to them, and to help them through their grief, however, adults are often reluctant to respond to children in grief. Sometimes it's due to their own grief, their own feeling of inadequacies, or simply not realizing how difficult grief is for children. All too often adults do not understand what a child needs after suffering a loss or how they can best provide the help that the child needs.

Grief can have long lasting effects into adult life if it is not resolved. Studies show that unresolved grief can result in depression, alcoholism, loneliness, accidents, anxiety, physical diseases, and suicide.

As a grief counselor, I have found very little material written about how to work with children in grief so I developed many of my own techniques, especially how to form support groups for grieving children. Over the years in private practice, I have collected information and techniques that have been useful in helping children through grief. I decided to write this book so that other professionals such as teachers, counselors, doctors, nurses, ministers, and social workers will have some techniques in helping a grieving child to understand what has happened, what they are feeling, and why.

This book was also written to help families, teachers and friends who are in the position to help a child through grief. For this reason, I chose to make this book more practical than technical. I want laymen to be able to apply it to their everyday lives. I have purposely omitted statistics, technical terminology, and results of recent research studies.

In this book I discuss what to teach a child about death, how and what to tell the child, about children and funerals, a child's understanding of death, normal grief reactions, how to develop and facilitate support groups for children, tools to use for facilitating insights and communications, the use of art with children, and the last chapter was written especially for parents. Also, throughout the book I try to give examples of the children that I have worked with and how they have come to understand and cope with their grief.

I hope that this book will give families and professionals encouragement that a grieving child can be helped and can do well in life. They can adjust and grow from the experience to become people with great inner strength.

All grief must not be thought of as being awful nor destructive. The world would be worse without it. If no person's life were significant enough to cause weeping and if the measure of our years on earth were nothing, then we would not be "real" human beings. Profound grief is preceded by deep love which gives life meaning.

In her book, "The Velveteen Rabbit," Margery Williams gives us some idea of what it means to be "real." The rabbit asks the wise old skin horse what it means to be "real." The skin horse replies, "Real isn't how you are made. It's a thing that happens to you. When a child loves you for a long, long time, not just to play with, but REALLY loves you, then you become Real."

"Does it Hurt?" asked the Rabbit.

"Sometimes," said the Skin Horse, for he was always truthful. "When you are Real you don't mind being hurt."

"Does it happen all at once, like being wound up," he asked, "or bit by bit?"

"It doesn't happen all at once," said the Skin Horse. "You become. It takes a long time. That's why it doesn't often happen to people who break easily, or have sharp edges, or who have to be carefully kept. Generally, by the time you are Real, most of your hair has been loved off, and your eyes drop out and you get loose in the joints and very shabby. But these things don't matter at all, because once you are Real you can't be ugly, except to people who don't understand."

"The Boy's Uncle made me Real," he said. "That was a great many years ago; but once you are Real you can't become unreal again. It lasts for always."

Acknowledgements

I want to thank my husband, Paul, for his patience with me and with this project. A very special thanks to my friend, Jan Kelley, for her many hours of typing this book, her loving criticism, and for her continual encouragement and prayers. Lastly, I want to thank the many children that I have grown to know and love during their grief. They have had the courage to deal with their grief and to grow from it.

1

UNDERSTANDING DEATH

Children's education about death should begin by explaining the natural part of the cycle of life—that all things (plants, animals, and people) are born, grow, live, and die. Farm children see the cycle of life and death in animals, crops, trees, and flowers; but today's city children have little awareness of such a cycle. Teaching about the life cycle, which can begin as early as one year of age, will set the tone for their understanding of death and allow the children's first questions. How the parents respond to these questions will influence if the child sees death as a natural or unnatural part of living. Often without meaning to, we repress a child's natural attitude toward death because of our own fears and our culture's unwillingness to talk about death.

Deanna Edwards (1984) stresses the importance of teaching children about the scale of life. On one side of the scale is the "good" (birth, youth, comfort, health, and laughter) which we all want. On the other side of the scale of life is what we consider the "bad" (death, old age, pain, illness, and tears) which we fear and try to escape. We need to teach our children to deal with both sides of the scale because we can grow and find happiness in both. We need to let our children feel pain; not to fear it. We can program them to handle pain and to succeed in spite of it. Our society has the misconception that happiness is the absence of pain, and we often go too far in protecting each other. As parents, we attempt to run interference on pain for our children and to solve their problems. In teaching our children about death and grief, we need to teach them how to deal with pain.

Many times the first experience a child has with death is the death of a pet. The death of that pet is a profound experience for children because they transfer feelings of love and human qualities to a pet. In some instances, grief for a pet has excelled grieving over the death of a parent or loved one. I remember one eight-year-old boy that would not cry after his father died but cried when telling me about the death of his pet that had died several months before the death of his father.

It is healthy to discuss with the children that their pet has died and then have a small funeral service. Where it is permitted by law, a smaller pet could be buried in the backyard. Children can have an active role in the funeral services and learn from these events. Children need and are entitled to a period of grief so don't immediately replace their pet with another pet. They may begin to believe that people can be replaced after they have died. In acquiring a new animal, it is important to stress the importance of memories (e.g., "Even with a new pet, you can always remember the times that you shared with your old friend.").

Do not dispose of the pet and just pretend it ran away or replace it with a new pet hoping the child won't know the difference. Children do know the difference, and they will lose their trust in what you say. You would be causing your child to deny the reality of death, and they may choose never to accept death as a part of life.

Telling the Child

First, tell the child naturally and compassionately about the loss as soon as possible. Children know immediately when something is wrong by the tone of a group. Their anxiety is

1

compounded when they are asked to leave the room or when the whispering begins. When I saw a ten-year-old girl one year after her dad died, she was angry because no one had explained to her what was happening the day her dad died. She had carried that anger around with her for a year.

Unfortunately, many parents, in struggling with their own grief, may think that their children will not understand the tragic situation and in doing so, create a feeling of isolation. School personnel may further heighten the child's feelings of isolation by acting as if nothing significant had occurred when the child returns to class.

Hold or touch the child when telling them about their loss. Remember, it is more important what you do than what you say. Let them know that you are there for them and will take care of them.

Do not overwhelm the child with excessive detail nor talk down to the child as if he or she is incapable of understanding. Tell the child the simple facts without a gruesome, terrifying description. One eleven-year-old girl in my support group had been told how bloody the accident had been that killed her father. When asked to draw a nightmare, she drew a picture of herself drowning in blood. Also, when asked to show something of her father's, she brought his bloody tennis shoe from the accident. In telling the child, proceed slowly with patience and gentleness. Most authorities encourage a natural explanation of the cause of death (e.g., "The cancer killed Dad."). The explanation that the disease was incurable is easier to understand than a loving God who takes "daddies" away or who kills little children. If possible, begin talking to the child of things that he or she has experienced or noticed already (e.g., "You've noticed how sick Grandma has been lately.").

Use the word "died." Have you noticed how people don't die anymore? They just "pass on," "pass away," "perish," "expire," "go away," "are lost," or "depart." These words get in the way of the child's understanding of death when they are attempting to distinguish reality from a world of fantasy. Tell the child the person will never return and that the person will be buried in the ground. Mention that the person can not breath, hear, see or move.

Do not tell the child that his loved one is sleeping because it heightens a child's fear of going to sleep at night. Some children actually struggle to remain awake, fearful they might go off to the deceased's type of "sleep" or that they might be put in a box and be put into the ground. Don't tell a sibling that his brother or sister went to live with God because he or she was good. You may find a reversal in behavior of an ordinarily obedient child who in no way is ready to be good and be taken from his parents to live with God.

If you tell the child that their loved one has "gone on a long journey" or is "lost," the child will continue to look for that loved one or may feel their loved one has abandoned him without saying "goodbye." They might then react with anger and resentment because their loved one really didn't care about them in the first place. If you say, "God wanted your Mommy with Him," a child might wonder, "Don't I need Mommy more than God?" and thus hold a deep resentment toward God.

I believe that our teaching about death should be coupled with teaching about heaven. I find that children do better with the understanding that with death there is a transition from earth to heaven rather than a complete cessation of life. Be careful not to tell a child that the deceased is not really dead. Death is a reality which must be faced and dealt with both psychologically and spiritually. Christians accept the reality of death, and affirm the reality of resurrection. With children, do not overemphasize the latter without first allowing them to encounter the reality of death and their emotional responses to it.

Encourage the child to voice questions even if it is the same question over and over. Be completely honest and tell the child, "I don't know," if you don't. Do not teach children as if we have the final answers that they must accept, but that we can learn together and can help each other. Questions that a child is likely to ask are: "What is death?" "Why do people have to die?" "What happens to people when they die; where do they go?" A child who gets an answer without overtones of reproach or a hint of uneasiness can trust what is being told to him or her. Silence only deprives the child of the opportunity to share grief.

Children should be encouraged to tell us how they feel about death, what they think, what they know, and how we can help them.

Children and Funerals

After the funeral has been explained to the children on their level, the choice should be up to them if they want to attend. Advantages of going to the funeral are that the child will experience the reality of death, and there will be many people to share in his or her sorrow. This gives the child a sense of support and of belonging. If ignored, the child often feels that he has done something wrong. Explain how the body will look and what will happen in the services and at the cemetery. They may want to view the body, but don't force them. Also, make sure the casket is completely open. Children fear that the other half of the body is gone if they see only the upper portion of the body.

They may be taken to the funeral home early by someone they love and trust. The advantage of going early is that they will not be frightened by an adult mourner's hysterical outburst, and they can freely express their feelings and emotions. I know some pastors who have a small private service for the children at the funeral home, and it seems to work quite well.

Some children choose not to attend the funeral or wake, even of their own parent. They should not be admonished or made to feel guilty about this choice. You may want to tape the service for the child to listen to at a later date. Also, if possible, allow children to make their contribution to the family by helping around the house such as answering the phone or door. They need to be included in the family's sorrow and receive the support of others around them.

Children's Perceptions of Death

Grownups tend to believe that death is not a proper concern for children, yet children are forever asking questions about death—sometimes directly; sometimes indirectly. As adults, we often have trouble helping children handle their grief or talk about death. Sometimes the difficulty arises from our own unresolved feelings about death or because we are enmeshed in our own sorrow. Evading discussion with remarks that children are "too young" may bring a degree of false comfort to adults.

A child growing up today is all to aware of the reality of death. Even at a very young age, the child may be confronted with death through a pet being killed or losing a grand-parent. The picture of death occurs almost daily on television—a leader is assassinated or astronauts are blown up in a space shuttle.

There are several phases in the child's awareness of death; and the child's age, psychological development, and maturity determine his or her ability to grasp the concept of death.

Children *under the age of three* have little actual understanding of death. Death is an abstract concept to them and their reaction is often one of curiosity rather than concern. Their grief is usually a reaction to separation rather than death itself. Infants and toddlers experiment with the concept of "being" and "nonbeing" by playing games such as "peek-a-boo."

Even though the children at this age have few language skills to ask questions or to describe their feelings, I do believe they still can *experience* a tremendous sense of loss and grief. One young family I worked with had an 18-month-old baby. After her father died of cancer, she appeared to be looking for something that was lost and waited for him to return daily. Around the age of three when she became verbal, she began to ask questions she had kept bottled up inside her (e.g., "Where is Daddy?" "Why did he have to die?" "What is heaven like?" "Will Daddy come home?"). We have to be very careful not to underestimate what the loss may mean to the very young child.

Children between the ages of *three and five* tend to view death as temporary like a rose that dies in the winter but returns alive to bloom in the spring again. Death is like sleep; you are dead and then you are alive again. It is like taking a journey; you are gone and then you come back again. They may "play dead" but come back to life as they have seen actors do on television.

At this age it is difficult for the children to separate the real world from their world of imagination and fantasy. They have many fantasies about death, such as "dead people eat at night when no one can see them," or that "dead people walk around at night." They believe that death is improbable and escapable (e.g., "Death happens only to old people, and I'll never get old."). They see parents as being able to "fix" anything; even death.

Later in this stage, the children develop "magical thinking." They believe they have the ability to make things happen by simply thinking or wishing. Young children have unlimited faith in their ability to make things happen, simply by wishing, and in their ability to undo things at will. The little girl will make her mom dead because she said, "no more cookies," and then later will bring her mom back to life when she needs something else. Some children fear that they have caused a loved one's death because they wished them dead or because they were angry with that person.

At some point, they become very curious and ask many questions about death. Because of their limited frame of reference, questions like, "Where is Mommy?" and "When will she come back?" are difficult to answer. Because children do not understand death, they may react with intense anger and experience severe rejection. The most important reality is still the separation from the dead person.

Children between the ages of *six to nine* gradually realize that death is final but may not understand it as something that will happen to everyone; particularly to themselves. They are influenced more by peer discussion, formal education, and the media. They have less magical thinking and more reliance on reality.

Often you will find a child around this age developing more fears. They may have more nightmares, such as airplanes crashing into their house or tornadoes carrying them away.

4

Also, they may request that a night light be left on. Some children become exceedingly anxious over death and may see death associated with violence.

Children at this age group have a strong tendency to personify death; to imagine it as a separate person. They tend to see death as a distinct personality such as a living being that can move, a soul, death angels, a skeleton, a spirit, or the "boogie-man;" that real death is everywhere so no one can escape. In working with children, I have them draw death and almost all of the younger children draw death as a living being that snatches people (even when they seem to have a good concept of heaven and the person's soul). Also, children seem to be accustomed to thinking about death at evening (a connection between death and darkness).

Many children see death as bad because it stops people from living; and often, they see a relationship between sin and death (e.g., "If you are bad, you will die.").

Between the ages of six to nine, many children have an almost obsessive interest in death, and at times they sound morbid. They may develop an interest in cemeteries or caskets and what happens to a dead body (e.g., "Can I jump on the grave?" "How do you eat or sleep when you are dead?" "Will it hurt to be dead?"). It is their way of dealing with the reality of death.

Children between the ages of *ten and twelve* have a more logical concept of death. They view death as a natural part of life. They no longer have magical thinking nor do they personify death. Around the ages of nine and ten, the child begins to realize that death is inevitable and universal. Death will happen to them, too. These children have become more "social beings" so their questions relate to, "Who will take care of my friend now?" and "Who will help you?" Often, to protect themselves or hide their fear, they make fun of death by telling ghost stories or jokes about death.

As children approach *adolescence*, they are equipped with most of the intellectual tools necessary to understand both life and death in a logical manner. It can be understood in relation to "natural law," yet, at the same time, adolescents and even adults have childlike views of death. They "know" that death is inevitable and final, but most of their daily activities and actions are more consistent with the conviction that personal death is an unfounded rumor. To integrate the concept into their total view of life they must face its personal implications.

Adolescents sometimes attempt to defy death by taking unnecessary risks, such as in their games of "Chicken" and "Russian Roulette," reckless driving, drinking, drug use, acting out sexually, or delinquent behavior. Symbolically, they may be saying, "We have so much anxiety over death that we play with it." Underneath it all, they are seriously seeking the meaning of life and attempting to test the boundaries of both life and death.

These are all rough approximations with many variations, but they may prove valuable in your understanding of children and grief. Just remember that each child is unique and an individual in their understanding of death.

2

NORMAL GRIEF REACTIONS

Grief is a natural emotional response to loss. Grieving is as natural as crying when we hurt, sleeping when we are tired, eating when we are hungry, or sneezing when we have a cold. It is nature's way of healing a broken heart. Children, like adults, must be allowed to grieve in rhythm to his or her own character and personality.

There are certain things that will influence how a child will deal with grief. First, we must look at the child's own chronological age, maturity and psychological understanding of death. Each child has different conceptual skills to understand what is going on.

Another influence will be the child's own strengths and weaknesses. Does the child normally react to stress with humor, anger, or withdrawal? How has this child handled other crisis in his or her life?

The history of the child's previous relationship with the person who has died affects his or her reaction to the loss. If the deceased and the child were exceptionally close and that person provided security, the loss is naturally greater for the child than if the loss was a distant relative. If the deceased and child had a relationship with a lot of conflicts, the child's sorrow may be intensified by guilt feelings.

Circumstances or nature of the death (was the death expected or unexpected?) will influence the child's grief. If the loved one has been murdered or killed in an accident, the child probably will feel shock followed by anger or rage. If the child's loved one has been terminally ill, he or she may feel relieved that it is over. Also, if there has been an accident without a body recovered, the child may have a hard time dealing with the reality of death.

We need to look at how many concurrent crisis or stress events the child may be dealing with at this time. Is he or she dealing with multiple losses which can include other things besides the loss of a loved one? A child can grieve over the loss of a pet, not making a team or cheerleader, poor grades, moving out of a neighborhood, changes in school or church, loss of friends, loss of dreams or ideals, loss of trust or values, loss of health, loss of money, etc.

Religious beliefs taught by the family are another influence on the child's perception of the death. A child's faith in God and an afterlife can help him or her cope with the death, but at times religious and ethnic subcultures can be harmful if they do not permit the child to grieve openly or if they teach that a loving God kills people.

The openness of the family system itself will influence the child's grief. The child needs the comforting presence of adults whom she or he can trust and can rely on in a continuing relationship. It helps if the child has come from a reasonably secure environment, has received prompt and accurate information about what has happened, and has been allowed to participate in the family's grieving.

When you take into consideration all of the influences, it is difficult to discuss grief as happening in stages or phases. Each child is unique and not one of them progresses like another, nor do they fit into categories. Instead of discussing stages of grief, I would rather discuss a child's normal grief reactions. A child may show all of these grief reactions or they may show only one or two of them. Do not tell the child that he or she should be having these reactions, but use them as guidelines to see if the child is within the normal limits of grief.

Children not only experience grief at different depths and at different rates, but also experience grief for different lengths of time. It will usually vary from one year to three years before their grief is resolved.

Shock or Numbness

Like adults, children are often numbed or temporarily stunned by the news of the death. The impact of the death may take a few minutes or a few days to be realized. You may even observe a child reacting casually after he or she has been told that a parent has died. One nine-year-old boy asked if he could go to the movies with a friend after being told that his father had died. Parents can easily misinterpret this delayed reaction. A parent may believe that the child did not love the deceased parent or may think that the child does not need to grieve. People around the child often reinforce this initial response by telling others how well the child is doing, how mature he or she is, or what a help the child has been to the rest of the family. These verbal and nonverbal messages can make it difficult later for the children to express their grief openly.

Shock is the body's physical denial and protection. The body system temporarily shuts down, sometimes to the point that the child is unable to cry. The child may even laugh or appear quite calm. Shock is like a protective bubble or cocoon around the child. Information begins to seep through little holes in the protective bubble as the child is able to deal with some of the reality of the death.

Denial

Some children are afraid to let down their emotional defenses and will deny that the person has died. He or she may be saying, "I don't believe it. It didn't happen. It is just a dream. Mommy will come back." Usually the lack of response signifies that the child has found the loss too great to accept and goes on pretending secretly that the person is still alive. Sometimes in dreams, the child senses the presence of the lost person so convincingly that it seems impossible the person is really away.

Denial can be expressed in several ways. The child may refuse to talk about the person that died or may shake his head "no" when you want to discuss the death. The child may act extra good to see if the parent will return (e.g., "If I am good, maybe my parent will return."). The child may deny that the parent ever existed or deny the importance of the person, especially if they feel that the absent parent has rejected them. One nine-year-old boy repeatedly said to me that he didn't care that his dad died because he didn't love his dad anyway. The mother told me that the dad had been a good dad. As long as the son continued to deny his love for the dad, he wouldn't have to feel the pain of that loss.

Panic or Alarm

After a loss of a parent, children are often frightened of what will happen to them now. There is a sense of vulnerability because the protector is gone. "Who will take care of me?" "Suppose something happens to my other parent?" "Who will get me the things that I need?"

They are apt to feel as if their world has come to an end and their own life is over. It is important for the surviving parent, a relative, or a close friend to reassure the child that they will look out for her, that they will be able to provide for her needs, and that they will be there to listen and to answer questions. The parent may need to say, "My health is fine. I will take care of you. There is enough money for food and toys."

A child may describe panic or alarm as a sore throat, tightness in the chest, or as having difficult in breathing. They may show signs of having an "anxiety" attack. Children have a difficult time labeling their feelings and often will say; "I have a funny feeling in my stomach but don't know why," "I feel weird and strange," or "I have mixed-up feelings, and I don't know what they are."

Fears

A child that has had a loss will have to deal with many fears. Fears about themselves dying may be stimulated by a parent's death, and they may fear that they will die the same way their loved one died. A boy may become preoccupied with the physical symptoms that terminated the life of his father. He may transfer the symptoms to himself in a process called identification. "I feel like Daddy when he died; I have a pain in my chest." A child may become oversensitive or react with unusual intensity to injuries or imagined injuries if someone they love died of an accident. Also, if one child dies, the other child may be reluctant and anxious about going places because of separation anxiety.

Participants in the children support groups developed this list of fears they have had since their loved one died:

- I won't ever see my loved one again.
- The world will come to an end because of war.
- I might die.
- Monsters might get me.
- Dead people will not stay buried but will walk around or will be on top of the ground.
- I might not get to heaven.
- Friends might treat me differently since my father died.
- Someone might break into the house; especially at night.
- I'm afraid of the nightmares that I have.
- Mother can't drive as safely as Dad did.
- I'm afraid to come home to an empty house after school.
- I'm afraid of the dark.
- My mother might start crying and then fall apart.
- No one will take care of me like Mom did.
- I won't make good grades in school.

One seven-year-old boy described how he put his favorite stuffed animal outside his door for protection at night since his dad was not there to protect him.

Fears often are revealed in the child's dreams or nightmares, and almost all children have nightmares following the death of a loved one. A common thread in most of their nightmares is of monsters.

Anger

Children do experience anger when a loved one dies. Their anger may be focused on God for taking their loved one, on the dead person for abandoning them, or on themselves if they feel that they have in any way caused the death. Many young children harbor fantasies that they are responsible for the death in the family. That is, if one wishes someone harm, the belief will bring results. Anger is also due to the unfairness of the situation because dreams are broken. One twelve-year-old boy said, "I am mad because it is unfair that God took my mother, and now I can't have a happy home like other children." An eighteen-year-old girl was angry at her father for his past behavior. He had been an alcoholic until he learned of his terminal disease. After he sobered up, she found out how nice her father could be and became very angry that he had wasted seven years of their relationship.

Children's anger may not be expressed toward the true target, but may be displaced or focused on someone or something that is less threatening. The child may express anger toward siblings, teachers, objects, the surviving parent for still being alive, or anyone who seemingly could have prevented the loss, (e.g., "My dad died because the doctor gave him the wrong medicine," or "Mother didn't take proper care of him."). Children also might make adults their target for anger if the adult seems to be pushing the child to accept the loss.

Anger is often not recognized but irritation, frustration, and annoyance may be shown. Observe if the child is slamming doors, kicking objects, or yelling a lot. There may be overpowering rage underneath what you are observing. One seven-year-old boy was ready to fight anyone. He often said, "I can beat up anyone I want to."

Anger can be a part of hurt. "Anger" has the same root as "anguish," but often we do not treat an angry child as a child in anguish. Instead we get upset with the child for showing any kind of anger. We say things like, "You really shouldn't be angry at God," or "You really don't mean that you are glad your sister died." One nine-year-old boy told me that he had been angry when his father was dying of cancer but his mother would never allow him to express this anger. He stated, "Being angry is not acceptable at my house." When asked what he did with his anger, he said, "My throat gets sore, and sometimes I feel like someone has their fingers around my throat." Some children will turn their anger into physical symptoms such as sore throats, headaches, tightness of muscles, and clenched fists.

Children usually feel guilty about their anger because they have been told that "nice children do not get angry." Few can admit their anger; much less cope with it. Healing begins when the child can disclose his or her anger to a tolerant and sympathetic listener. Children need to be reassured that anger like other grief reactions will be resolved when they get their feelings out in the open and deal with them; that they will not be punished or condemned for their feelings, and also, that God understands their outburst and does not punish them for it.

Support group participants developed this list of what they have been angry about since their loved one died:

- Angry at the lady that killed my dad in the accident.
- That my sister wouldn't cry after our dad died.
- That I wasn't home when my father died.
- That others wouldn't tell me what happened for a long time.
- That I wasn't in the car with my dad when he had the accident. I could have prevented it by telling him to be careful.

9

- That Dad didn't kiss me good night before he died.
- That I didn't get to do some things that I wanted to during my brother's/father's illness.
- That I am now in charge of my sister and brothers, and they don't listen to me.
- That there are too many things to do now.
- That Dad doesn't listen since Mom died.
- That my parent doesn't respect my rights.
- That parents blame us when things aren't going right.
- Mad at the dragon that took Dad away because I'm not suppose to be mad at God or my Dad.

Guilt/Regrets

In working with younger children, you may want to use the term "regrets" instead of guilt because some have difficulty in understanding the concept of guilt. Children do have to deal with some degree of guilt or regrets so don't minimize it or tell them that they shouldn't be feeling that way. Let them get it out in the open. Unresolved guilt, whether "normal" or "neurotic" may be harmful physically and mentally.

Rosen (1984-85) found that guilt is a commonly reported reaction to the loss of a sibling: including guilt for being alive when the sibling had died, for having been well when the sibling was ill, for having wished the sibling dead at some time in their relationship, etc.

In grief we find three kinds of guilt: 1) Survivor syndrome—where the person will ask, "Why did they die instead of me?" 2) Real guilt—due to doing or not doing something while the family member is alive. "I acted out of carelessness which caused the accident." Also, some guilt is due to unexpressed anger that the child may be having. In dealing with real guilt, you need to find ways that he or she can learn to forgive themselves. I sometimes ask the child, "What does it take for you to be able to forgive yourself?" 3) Imaginary guilt—thoughts can kill. "My brother died because I fought with him and wished he was dead."

Imaginary or unrealistic guilt usually stems from a situation which was uncontrollable. This type of guilt is irrational and must be discussed. Sometimes their imaginary guilt is due to lack of knowledge or incomplete thinking. We may need to help them complete their thinking. A child's assumption of responsibility may be characterized by a preoccupation with the "should haves." At times like this, adults may need to share their own confusion and guilt about the situation with them. A child saw his younger brother hit by a car while they were outside playing and kept saying, "I should have watched him closer." Taking the child in her arms, his mother said, "I, too, wish I had watched him closer and that I could do it over again, but this is a choice we do not have, and even though we feel guilty it is not our fault."

One seven-year-old support group participant paced continually when talking about his dad's death. He paced around the room pointing at the other children saying, "I hope you take better care of your 'dads' than I did. If I ever get a new dad, I will take better care of him." The young boy felt totally responsible for his dad's death because he had been angry with his dad a few weeks before he was killed in a car accident. The father had been teaching the boy to ride a bicycle, and the boy was slow catching on. The dad became angry and put the bike up in the garage making the boy so angry that he yelled "I hate you" wishing at the time that his dad was dead. A few weeks later the boy's wish came true.

10

Some guilt/regrets that the children have mentioned in the support groups:

- My brother's/father's death might have been my fault.
- I wasn't always nice to my loved one.
- I wish I could have been home when my dad died.
- I called my parent mean names when I was mad.
- I should have been able to prevent the accident.
- I was embarrassed how my father looked after receiving treatments for cancer.
- I got mad at my loved one.
- I didn't tell my parent how much I loved him or her before he or she died.
- I didn't get to spend time alone with my mother before she died of cancer because there were always other adults around. I wanted to tell her some things.
- Once I got so angry that I hit my mother.

One young boy told how he was given some of the Christmas gifts meant for his father because his father was too sick to have them, and his father died shortly after Christmas. The boy felt like he had cheated his father by taking the gifts.

Idealization

Sometimes when a child has lost a parent they tend to idealize that parent; they become obsessed with the parent's good qualities, (e.g., "How dare you say anything against my Mommy! She was perfect."). The falsification is out of keeping with the parent's real life and character. The child may even assume some of the mannerisms or characteristic traits of the deceased by walking and talking like that parent. The child may even wish that the surviving parent had died instead; especially when the parent has to do all of the disciplining. This can lead to angry outbursts or guilt.

Encourage the child to not only remember the good qualities of that dead parent but also a weakness or two that made the parent human. It helps remove the pressure the child has put on himself or herself to be perfect and to follow in the parent's footsteps. They need to have a balanced view of that parent.

Tears

Children feel sad after a loss, and it is normal to shed tears when one is sad. Tears are a natural part of grief, and they are needed to relieve stress. Research now shows that not all tears are the same. Tears resulting from sadness, anger, fear, and joy are chemically different from those induced by onions and other irritants. We all feel better after crying because we may be removing from the body chemicals that build up as a result of emotional stress. When we cry, we give off protein and albumin which if kept in the body becomes toxic poisoning.

We need tears to wash away the gray tensions of our soul and when we do cry, it does not require an apology nor an explanation. So often in our society today, no one is given permission to cry. If you do cry, people consider you close to a breakdown, to losing it, or you are falling apart. Tears are a human right.

At the same time, I have seen children who do not cry because they are afraid of losing control—once they start they may never be able to stop. Sometimes they need permission to cry and the reassurance that someone will be there to help them regain control again. Also, a child may not cry because he or she feels very protective toward a parent. "If I cry, I might upset Mom, and I don't want her to hurt anymore." One nine-year-old boy told me that he had not cried since his father's death a year ago because his father used to laugh at him when he would cry. "Big boys don't cry."

Relief at Death

Sometimes children are relieved that the person has died; especially if the deceased had a long illness. The child hopes things will finally return to normal. "Now I can go places that I want and I couldn't before because of Mommy's illness." The child may also be relieved that the deceased parent's restrictions and expectations for them are gone. This relief reaction can later lead to guilt or shame; especially if adults are shocked and harsh with the child for sharing this with them. Also, a child who has gone through anticipatory grieving may have already completed some of his or her actual grief.

Physical Reactions

There will be a physical adaptation to the loss. At first, there may be an increase in heart rate, sweating, and rapid breathing. Later, they are prone to more infections—especially colds, sore throats, and ear infections. The "biology of grief" appears to produce major perturbations in the respiratory, central nervous, and hormonal systems and may substantially alter functions of the heart, blood, and immune or infection fighting systems as well. You may see skin rashes, tightness of muscles, burning on urination, and the child having a low energy level. One thirteen-year-old boy had several rashes during the time I saw him, and the medical doctor could not find a reason for the rashes except stress.

Children in grief may eat all of the time to fill up their emptiness. One ten-year-old girl told me that she ate when she was lonely. Other children may not eat at all and hoard the food so no one can take it away from them.

Grieving children are more prone to accidents. They become careless because they are preoccupied with death. In one family after the father was killed, two of the three small children broke their arms within a few days of one another. Also, one fourteen-year-old boy broke his fists and another deeply cut his finger two different times.

Disorganized

Grieving takes so much of the child's energy that little is left to attend to other aspects of living. It will be difficult for the child to concentrate and to get organized. Daily routines such as brushing teeth or combing hair may be forgotten and making decisions are exhausting. School may become a problem (for up to two years) after their loss.

Regression

Regression, especially among younger children, is common. They may regress in one area of their life but not in all areas. The child may wet the bed, soil his pants, suck his thumb, have temper tantrums, pull at his hair, bite nails, and whine or cling excessively. He might request a night light on or request to sleep with the parent(s).

Low Self-Esteem

It is common for children to go through a period where they lose all confidence and think very little of themselves. Low self-esteem can be due to their own vulnerability, to not having control over a situation, or to some unresolved guilt. A vast majority of children assume that they were in some way responsible for their loss. Children may decide that "I was so bad that God took my parent from me" or "I was so unlovable that my parent didn't want to be around me." These self-imposed labels "bad" and "unlovable" deal the child's self-esteem a terrible blow from which many children are slow to recover. When one mother told her son she loved him after his father died, he would reply, "I don't love me." He shared with me that he did what he wanted to because he felt no one cared anyway.

Loneliness/Yearning

A feeling of loneliness occurs often in grief. One eight-year-old girl described it as "an empty feeling in my tummy." Children do yearn for their lost loved one and in one recent study (Fox, 1984-85), children identified a variety of points at which they most missed the family member during the previous year; times when they needed the relative's help or friendship, on holidays (especially Thanksgiving, Christmas, and Easter), on the dead person's birthday; and on the day of the week when the relative died. The other times during the year when they have found themselves remembering the dead family member include when they are doing things they used to do with the relative, when they see a dead sibling's friends, and when they go to bed. I find that children have a difficult time around the calendar date of when their loved one died.

A family of four shared they missed and yearned for their mother's cooking, her being there when they got home from school, her holding them when they were sick or hurt, her good sense of humor, and her helping them with school work.

Yearning is the reaction in grief that stays with us throughout life. A young woman who loses her mother as a child will often yearn to have her mother present at her wedding. A young man may yearn to have his father share in the birth of the first grandson.

Depression and Apathy

A child usually deals with some degree of depression during grief. Sometimes it is the result of unexpressed emotions such as anger or guilt. The child may be thinking, "Will life ever be worth living again?" Though rarely acted upon, suicidal thoughts exist in some children. They may be thinking about rejoining their lost loved one.

Children with depression may have slowed thinking and actions, physical complaints, bland expression, problems with sleeping or sleep a great deal, and may weep at inappropriate times. Also, you may see withdrawal or decreased socialization often due to the fact that they feel as if their friends do not understand what they are going through. They may want to escape into books or television. One twelve-year-old boy after losing both parents escaped to his room with his computers.

It is very important to be alert about the possibility of depression, but we also need to be careful to distinguish between depression and sadness. In our society, the word depression has tended to replace the word sadness. We rarely perceive or verbalize sadness, but instead claim one as being depressed. Some children are mistakenly treated for depressive illness while the sadness and the need to grieve go unrecognized.

Searching, Hyperactivity, or Restlessness

A restless child may walk into a room, look around, and then leave again. He may pace or his eyes may continuously roam when you talk to him because he is subconsciously looking for what has been lost, or he may go over and over the events leading to the death trying to make sense out of the death. He will probably ask, "Why?" over and over which he needs to do even if he doesn't find answers.

Sometimes hyperactivity can be denial. The child (especially adolescents) keeps busy to avoid thinking about what has happened. This frantic activity has the additional benefit of warding off awareness of reality. Searching behavior may continue for months, changing from the early aimless motion to a later filling up of every spare moment with activity. This leads to the danger of the child becoming physically and emotionally exhausted.

Changes in Roles

Bereaved children must cope with the changes in their day-to-day lives which often include changes in their roles and responsibilities. They may have to make the shift from two parents to one which may mean less attention from the surviving parent. The widowed parent may be emotionally unavailable to them or physically unavailable if working long hours. There also may be a change in the amount of income if a parent dies. It can mean giving up activities that take extra money or can result in a change of neighborhood, school, and friendships.

A father is often an important symbol of authority even if the mother does most of the disciplining. After a father dies, children may show less respect for her knowing that the father cannot intervene. At the loss of a mother, the father may become overwhelmed by the many demands of parenting, homemaking, and may have a difficult time nurturing his children. Also, a parent may become overly strict because they don't have the other parent to balance out the situation with humor and compassion. Some widowed parents may have difficulty setting limits because they feel badly for their children's loss.

The children may have to assume a greater emotional and functional role in the family. Often a widowed parent looks to the children for nurturance or for help in decision making. Older children may be given responsibility of the younger children. One fourteen-year-old boy shared with me his anger and resentment about having to be responsible for cooking, housecleaning, babysitting, and helping younger children with homework after his mother died. He felt overwhelmed by all of it. If not careful, too much responsibility can tie a child to the family indefinitely.

One eighteen-year-old girl felt responsible for her younger brother after their father died. Since her mother was working, she was home more and became aware of her brother taking drugs. She carried this burden for quite awhile before sharing it with her mother.

14

Resolved Grief

With the right type of support, children do learn to work through their grief and often become a stronger person for it. Children from single-parent homes can do well in life. One study found 40% of eminent scientists had lost one parent through death. Children can learn to integrate losses into their personality. They will never become their "old self" again but will learn to redefine roles and their self-image. The child can reorganize herself or himself to get on with life.

If you have been helping a child through the grieving period, there will probably be no clear ending to signify the child's passage from active grief into resolved grief. There are some healthy signs to observe for in children:

- Positive self-esteem will be restored.
- They will focus on the present instead of the past and will make plans for the future.
- They will make new friends.
- School grades will improve.
- They will be able to give encouragement to others.
- They may become more verbal about death and feelings without fear of being thought of as different.
- Tears are less frequent.
- They will be able to feel warm affections for others.
- They will be able to return to normal activities.
- Humor returns, and they are able to laugh again.
- They will be able to give human qualities to their deceased loved one.
- They will be able to do some problem solving and make some decisions again.

Trouble Signs

One eleven-year-old girl showed several of the trouble signs one year after her father was killed. She had not been able to attend her father's funeral; she had been forced to move from one state to another; she had changed schools twice within a few months; and no one seemed to have the time to listen to this child. The school had found several notes the girl had written about wanting to be dead. When I saw her, she had disassociated herself from any feelings about her father, and she refused to feel any pain. She had a blank expression on her face and did not want to talk about her father nor remember him. She acted out in the sessions and made inappropriate comments. She stated that when she got unhappy she felt like burying herself, and she didn't plan on being around by the age of eighteen. She also said that when she got mad, she would scream, kick things, or argue with television commercials.

A child will give clues or signs that he or she is in trouble; that grief is not progressing as it should be. Observe for:

- Problems in school such as a drop in grades or behaving destructively toward others.
- Delinquent behavior (acting out in school or at home).
- Self-destructive behaviors such as excessive use of alcohol or drugs.
- Acting out sexually.
- Slamming doors.

- Smashing things or loud cursing.
- No emotions or a loss of feelings.
- Overactivity.
- Psychosomatic conditions (may acquire the symptoms of their lost loved one).
- Personality changes (e.g., may think everyone is against them).
- Retreating from social activities or becoming isolated.
- Talking or giving hints that they are thinking about suicide.
- Giving away his possessions.
- May remain angry or depressed.
- May become unusually vulnerable to new separations.
- May underachieve.

Grief becomes abnormal if it prevents the person from resuming normal activities. For many children, additional help is needed before they show positive integration of their loss.

3

SUPPORT GROUPS

The purpose of a children's support group is to help bereaved children learn ways of coping with loss and the resulting pain. The purpose of the group is not to achieve resolution of grief, but rather to give the children the skills and support to continue to work toward resolution of their grief. Also, it helps children to know that others are willing to listen and to know that they aren't alone in how they are feeling. By hearing others express similar emotions, children often recognize the normality and universality of these emotions. The group's nonjudgmental acceptance of the varying emotions encourages the individual's acceptance of them.

The group should be both educational and supportive in nature. Each session is to focus on a specific topic, and discussion is encouraged. Topics for discussion can include: "Feelings," "What Is Death," "Grief Reactions," "Remembering," "Dealing with Feelings," "Taking Care of Yourself," "Changes in Roles and Needs," "Parents Participation, Evaluation, and Closure."

Groups will meet with a facilitator and are limited to four to eight children. The group meets weekly for six to eight weeks depending on how you want to set up your program. Each session runs one and a half hours with the last session sometimes lasting two hours.

It is difficult to have a good cohesive group if there is a wide gap in the children's ages. The group will be influenced by the child's chronological and psychological understanding of death. The groups work best if broken down: 6 through 9, 8 through 10, 10 through 12, or 13 through 16. If you mix younger children with older children, there are problems of the younger ones not understanding what the older ones are saying or going through. Also, the older children don't always have patience with the younger children and may have a tendency to make fun of them by teasing.

First, meet with the parents (parent or guardian) of each child and explain what you will be doing in the group. Stress the importance of each child attending all sessions, and ask the parents to encourage the child to do the homework assignments on their own. When it is completed, they are not to see the assignment unless the child wants to share it. Inform the parents that sometimes children will appear to regress or be preoccupied during the weeks of the sessions because it takes a great deal of energy to share and to work on grief, but at the end they will be stronger for it. Encourage them to attend the last session with their child.

Confidentiality of the group needs to be discussed with the parents. Parents will not be told what goes on in the group by the facilitator without the child's permission. If there is a problem with the child that the parents need to know, then the facilitator needs to work very hard to get the child's permission to discuss it with his or her parents. Of course, the children can share what they want to with their parents.

You can get a child into a support group too soon. They may still be in shock or if it has been a long terminal illness, they may be feeling relief that their loved one has died. If this happens, the child has not faced the reality of the death and is not aware of the issues they will have to deal with at a later date. From my experience, I have seen that it usually takes children longer to get into their grief than it does adults. They seem to be in denial longer, and they often don't have the conceptual skills to understand fully what their loss will mean. I would rather not take a child into the group if it has been less than three months since the loss and would prefer that it has been six to twelve months after the loss. I have found that children have benefited from the group even if it has been a year and a half after their loss.

Many bereaved children were not certain that they needed or wanted to participate in the support group. They all said later after the group had begun that they thought it would just be children sitting around crying. They didn't know that it would be helpful and also fun. Most children come because of the encouragement of their parents. Occasionally, a child will request help.

Some children may cry during the sessions. Emotional release is natural and desirable. No one should be admonished or ridiculed for crying. Rather than saying to the child, "You mustn't cry," it is better to say, "I could cry, too," or "We cry when we feel pain." This lets the child know that crying is one way human beings have to recover from hurts and that adults cry at times also.

This chapter gives guidelines for seven separate sessions in a support group. These are just guidelines and can be adapted to meet the group's needs. The facilitator needs to take into consideration the type of losses, ages and number of the children, personalities, type of families they come from, and problems the children may be having at that specific time.

Observations About the Groups

I find that children (7 through 14) are verbal and willing to share. While one child is talking, I am aware of those that are nodding their heads in agreement. I point it out to those children to encourage further comment and to encourage their involvement in the group.

The support group opens up communications that carry over to the family outside the group. As one mother wrote in a thank-you note, "My daughter always looked forward to your group and would relate very openly to me some of her experiences. It provided a base of awareness for further communication."

In having the children evaluate their group, they all agreed that children suffering a loss should have a support group. The greatest benefit was hearing that other children were dealing with the same issues they were, and it made them feel "more normal." Also, they feel safer sharing these things with the group than with parents because they didn't want to upset parents who are already upset. It is hard to share with friends because their friends often see them as different. The one negative thing they said about the group is that after seven weeks it was over too soon and that they might not see some of their newly made friends again.

One of the positive things about the groups that I hadn't anticipated was that the parents often develop a support group among themselves while waiting for their children. It might even be possible to have a facilitator that could work with just the parents in a separate group.

18

Session I
Children's Support Group
Feelings

Purposes:

1. To establish rapport through gentle, nonprobing techniques.
2. To identify different feelings and how one's body reacts to each feeling.
3. To share how they are feeling at that moment.

Materials Needed:

1. Game: "Find Someone Who" (Exercise 1).
2. Art paper.
3. Crayons, pencils or magic markers.
4. Refreshments.
5. Name tags.
6. 5 sheets of paper for each child with one feeling (happy, lonely, scared, mad, sad) written across the top of each piece.

Expectations/Rules:

1. Purpose of the support group and what each session will be about.
2. Projects the group will be doing.
3. Confidentiality among the children.
4. Parents will not be told what goes on in the group without the children's permission, but the children are free to share their own thoughts and feelings with their parents if they so desire.
5. Children are encouraged to participate but not pressured to do so. The group is a safe place for sharing.
6. It is important to show respect for one another and not to laugh at each other or interrupt one another.
7. Homework assignments will be given, but they are not required to be shared. Grades are not given.
8. It is important that children attend all seven sessions.
9. Location of restrooms.

Do:

1. Each child introduces self; tells something they like about themselves, and what their loss is.
2. Play the game "Find Someone Who" (Exercise 1).
3. Next, using the prepared sheets on feelings, have each child draw how his or her face looks when they have a specific feeling (e.g., happy, lonely, scared, mad, sad).
4. On the art paper, have them draw how they are feeling at that moment.

Sharing Period:

1. Let the children share their pictures.

19

2. Discuss each of the specific feelings and how the body feels with each emotion.
3. Let the children share their picture on how they are feeling at that moment.
4. Discuss what other feelings they can think of (e.g., mixed-up, silly, embarrassed, helpless, shame, guilt or regrets, etc.).

Refreshments

Snacks may be popcorn, crackers, cookies, ice cream bars, juice, etc.

Assignments:

1. Draw a picture of how your family was before the death.
2. Do worksheet "Feeling Good" (Exercise 2).
3. Bring your favorite possession to share with the group next week.

Try to share hugs with each child before they leave unless they are uncomfortable with it.

Session II
Children's Support Group
What is Death

Purpose:

1. To increase the child's understanding about what happens in death.
2. To let the child know that what he or she is feeling or thinking is normal.

Materials Needed:

1. A warm-up exercise (e.g., "If you could be anyone you would like to be, who would it be and why?").
2. Art paper.
3. Crayons, pencils or magic markers.
4. Refreshments.
5. A short book about death (see Appendix D).
6. Tissues.

Do:

1. Take up assignment "Feeling Good" (Exercise 2).
2. Warm-up exercise.

Sharing Period:

1. Let each child share his favorite possession.
2. Let each child share her picture of how her family was before the death, and encourage her to discuss the relationship she had with her loved one.
3. Let each child draw a picture of what he thinks death is, and then tell about his picture. (When finished, I sometimes share pictures other children have drawn to encourage further discussion.)

Refreshments

Do:

1. Read a short story about death.
2. Give the children time to ask questions or make comments while you are reading.

Assignments:

1. Do worksheet "Grief Reactions" (Exercise 3).
2. Do worksheet "Changes" (Exercise 4).

Session III
Children's Support Group
Grief Reactions

Purposes:

1. To develop an understanding of the grief process.
2. To understand the range of emotions that occur after the death of a loved one, express some of these emotions, and learn to accept these emotions in oneself and others.

Materials Needed:

1. Art paper.
2. Crayons, pencils or magic markers.
3. Refreshments.
4. Tissues.

Sharing Period:

1. Let the children share their assignments "Grief Reactions" (Exercise 3) and "Changes" (Exercise 4).
2. Have each child fill out the true or false worksheet "Grief" (Exercise 5) and then discuss.
3. Share with the children normal grief reactions and discuss some of the reactions they may have had or may have in the future.

Refreshments

Assignments:

1. Bring something of your loved one to share with the group.
2. Make a list of the things you liked about your loved one.

Session IV
Children's Support Group
Remembering and Dealing with Feelings

Purposes:

1. To develop a realistic memory of the person(s) who died.
2. To give them a chance to tell about and remember their loved one.
3. To let the children identify their own fears, anger, and guilt and to let them know that these feelings are normal in grief.
4. To help them find constructive ways to deal with these feelings.

Materials Needed:

1. Art paper.
2. Chalk board or easel.
3. Crayons, pencils or magic markers.
4. Refreshments.
5. Tissues.

Sharing Period:

1. Let each child share what they brought of their loved one.
2. Let them share their list of what they liked about their loved one.
3. Encourage each child to share something they didn't like about their loved one.

Refreshments

Do:

1. Have the children draw a picture of a nightmare they have had since their loved one died. If they say that they haven't had one, have them draw any dream they can remember. Let the children share their drawings.
2. As a group, let the children make a list of their fears, a list of their guilt feelings or regrets, and a list of what they are angry about. Write the lists on a blackboard or easel.
3. Discuss how having these feelings are normal and discuss "Constructive Ways of Dealing with Your Feelings" (Exercise 6).

Assignments:

1. Do worksheet "Support" (Exercise 7). Discuss with the children what the terms support, helper, hinderer, and influence mean.
2. Do worksheet "I Believe in My Abilities" (Exercise 8).

Session V
Children's Support Group
Taking Care of Yourself

Purposes:

1. To recognize one's own need for help during grief.
2. To assess one's own strengths.
3. To identify some ways of coping.
4. To learn how to reach out to others and ask for help.
5. To learn where else they can obtain support if they need it.

Materials Needed:

1. Art paper.
2. Crayons, pencils, or magic markers.
3. Chalk board or easel.
4. Refreshments.
5. Tissues.

Sharing Period:

1. Have children share worksheet "Support" (Exercise 7). Discuss what it means to have someone who is supportive then discuss other possible supportive resources.
2. Have the children share worksheet "I Believe in My Abilities" (Exercise 8), and discuss their own strengths.
3. Discuss "Taking Care of Yourself" (Exercise 9).

Refreshments

Do:

1. As a group have the children make a list of things parents can help them with. Do not put names by the statements, and get the children's permission to share this list with their parents the last session.

Assignments:

1. Do worksheet "Problem Solving" (Exercise 10).

Session VI
Children's Support Group
Changes in Roles and Needs

Purposes:

1. To recognize changes in roles and needs as part of grief.
2. To evaluate one's own changes (both loss and acquisitions).
3. To look at how their family is functioning as a unit.

Materials Needed:

1. Chalk board or easel.
2. Paper and pencils.
3. Refreshments.
4. Tissues.

Sharing Period:

1. Discuss worksheet "Problem Solving" (Exercise 10). Ask if they have had to deal with a problem that is not on the worksheet, and discuss possible solutions for that problem.
2. Have each child write down the responsibilities they have at home. Have them put a star by those that are new since their loved one has died, then let them share their list with one another.
3. Discuss the roles they have in the family. If it is group therapy with children from one family, have them look at who is the leader, compromiser, talker, listener, peacemaker, aggressor, sensitive one, critic, encourager, follower, parent, etc.
4. As a group, have them make a list of their needs that are not being met because of the death of their loved one. Share this at the last session with their parents.

Refreshments

Assignments:

1. Have them write to their parent about a problem they are having on worksheet "Letter" (Exercise 11).
2. Worksheet "Child of the Year" (Exercise 12)—have them write a paragraph about why they would be selected.
3. Issue an invitation for parents to come to the next meeting.

Session VII
Children's Support Group
Parent Participation, Evaluation, and Closure

Purposes:

1. To educate parents about children's grief reactions.
2. To share with the parents some of the needs the children have and ways they would like for the parents to help meet these needs.
3. To let the children see some of the changes in roles and responsibilities the parents have.
4. To discuss ways the family can help one another so that they can function more as a family unit.
5. To evaluate the effectiveness of the group.
6. To end the group in a manner that the family can call you if a problem arises.

Materials Needed:

1. Art paper.
2. Crayons, pencils, or magic markers.
3. Chalk board and easel.
4. Refreshments.
5. Bring group's lists of how the children's needs have changed and of how their parents can help them with their grief.
6. "Evaluation" (Exercise 13).
7. Tissues.

Sharing Period:

1. Take up assignments (not to be shared as a group because parents will be present).
2. Have each person (parents and children) draw how they see themselves now. Have each person tell about their picture.
3. Go over list of the children's needs and the list on how their parents can help them in grief. Give parents time to respond and to add what their needs are.
4. Have parents as a group make a list of how their roles and responsibilities have changed since their loved one has died.
5. Let the group make suggestions and share what they would like from one another so they could function better as a family unit.
6. After dismissing children to go to another room to complete "Evaluation" (Exercise 13), discuss with parents normal grief reactions and feelings their children *may* or *may not* have during grief.

Refreshments

Do:

1. Discuss briefly with the children and their parents what the group has meant to them.
2. Encourage children and parents to keep in contact if they have any questions, problems, or if they want to share something special that has happened to them.

4

COMMUNICATION TOOLS

It is often inappropriate to expect a young child to talk through his or her feelings because they are limited in their verbal skills and have immature cognitive processes. Most children do not reach the stage of formal operations in which problems are solved objectively by the process of hypothesis testing until the age of eleven or later.

Many children are also uncomfortable or unpracticed in talking about their feelings. When asked about their feelings, they may respond, "I don't know." They may not truly know, or it may be an easy answer that means, "I don't want to talk about it." Keep in mind that many children are unaccustomed to talking with adults other than family, close friends of the family, or teachers. Some children have never talked to adults who really listen and who try to understand their feelings so don't expect these children to accept you readily.

An excellent way to begin talking about feelings or about death with a child is to use activities or tools. I have found these to be useful in building communication, especially with younger children. As children mature and grow in their verbal and cognitive abilities, more and more of the help will likely be through direct conversation.

I have developed several activities and written material to enhance the communication between you and the child. These activities can also be used to assess the child's progress during grief, his or her understanding of death, and what problems or concerns he or she may be having. The purpose of assessment is to identify areas in which the child is not functioning effectively and to determine what factors might be contributing to the difficulty. The assessment process in working with children requires special knowledge and skill because the capabilities of children change markedly from year to year, and also, the challenges of grief depend in large measure on the significant adults in the child's life.

Worksheets

One way to facilitate insights and communications is by the use of worksheets. In Appendix D are examples of worksheets designed to help you know the child better, extend their own self-awareness and promote understanding of others. When choosing which worksheet to use, keep in mind the child's age, his or her maturity, and the skills the child may or may not have.

Feelings Worksheets (Exercises 2, 14-15) are designed to help the children identify their feelings, to help them become aware that it is okay to have these feelings, and to let you know what the child is feeling.

Getting To Know You Worksheets (Exercises 16 & 17) are designed to promote the child's understanding of self and your understanding of the child.

Self-Worth Worksheets (Exercises 8, 12, & 18) are designed to encourage the child to identify their own strengths and weaknesses, and to let them know that it is okay to feel good about themselves.

Problem-Solving Worksheets (Exercises 10, 11, 19 & 20) are designed to assess the child's skills in problem solving, to encourage the child to see one's self as a resource to solve problems, to help the child develop situational skills (what is going on around them and how they respond), and to help the child associate consequences with decisions and actions.

Relationships Worksheets (Exercises 7, 21 & 22) are designed to promote understanding of others, and to encourage the child to identify his or her support system.

Grief Reactions Worksheets (Exercises 3 & 5) encourage the child to identify their grief reactions and allows them to know that different feelings during grief are normal.

Remembering Worksheets (Exercise 23) encourage the child to remember their past and the good times they have had with their loved one who has died.

Games

Unstructured games allow the child to place his or her own meanings on the play and are, therefore, usually better than structured games. Also, structured games often require the adult to enter into competition with the child, and there must be a winner and a loser. In most instances, if the adult plays at his or her skill level, he or she will win, creating a failure experience for the child. If the adult lets the child win, there is the risk that the child will recognize the manipulation and the genuineness of the relationship will be lost. Taking all of this into consideration, I still occasionally use a structured game with a child that is having difficulty communicating because it can be a safe, relaxed time for the child to talk. I find putting a puzzle together is helpful, or you may want to use a commercial game about life where the child needs to answer some questions (e.g., The Ungame). One game that is my favorite to use is "Fish" described by Claudia L. Jewett (1982). For this game you need four or five sets of faces, usually including mad, happy, sad, scared, and lonely. Shuffle the cards and deal five to a person, then play the game like "Go Fish" except that when a pair is laid on the table the player with the pair must tell about a time he had that feeling.

Draw a Life Loop

With older children, have them draw a life loop of the high points in their life and of the low points in their life, then have them discuss how they felt at these high and low points and how they coped at those low times in their life. Encourage them to look at their strengths and help them to see how they can build on these strengths.

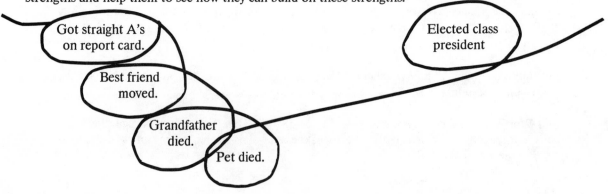

Play Therapy

Play therapy can be used to facilitate communications. A younger child is limited in her or his verbal skills and has difficulty verbalizing feelings of frustrations, love, anger, and guilt. The child may not be able to verbalize his or her emotions, but the child can act out his feelings. He crashes cars together, he hugs those that he loves, and he yells at or shoots the enemy so the introduction of play provides a means for communication that is natural for the child.

Play therapy provides a comfortable atmosphere in which constant conversation is not necessary. The child has the undivided attention of an adult and he or she has the freedom to express meaningful thoughts and feelings. It allows for learning and emotional release.

In the process of communication through play, there is some element of safety provided by the fact that the child is one step removed from real life. As a child acts out the death in the family using puppets or dolls, he or she may or may not directly describe the characters as his or her own family. The child can still explore how each member of the play family feels and growth can still occur. If on the other hand the child makes the connection with his or her real world, the helper may follow the child's lead.

In play therapy with children in grief, you may use either puppets, dolls, little play figures, clay, or a play telephone. Among the dolls, puppets, and little play figures, there should be males, females, adults, and children. The toys should be simple enough that the child can use his or her imagination in playing with them.

The adult can pretend with the child and then step back and make observations and help the child think about what has been happening. It helps if you reflect on the emotions and meanings that the play reveals. You can encourage the child to add some verbal expression to the process. Also, children benefit by hearing their feelings restated because they often need help in labeling their feelings.

One nine-year-old boy had been angry with the way his father had disciplined him. After his father died, he carried that anger with him into the grief, but he could not find the verbal words to describe what made him so mad. By the use of puppets he was able to play a father disciplining his son and then he played the son being disciplined by the father. The nine-year-old boy felt safe to express his anger toward the puppet and found himself yelling and very angry at the father puppet. It was the beginning of this boy openly admitting that he was angry.

Another young boy was very angry at the lady who killed his father in a drunken driving accident. He played himself as a puppet telling the lady puppet off and ended up beating on her. When she said she was sorry, he refused to believe her. He told her that the only way he would ever forgive her would be if she lost her driver's license and then went to jail. He then used one of the puppets to be God and told the lady that she would not be forgiven.

As children approach puberty, they begin to leave toys such as puppets and dolls behind, but pillows or punching bags can still be punched to express anger. Drawing, sculpturing, building with nails and hammer, or verbal role playing may be very useful activities.

Writing

Writing can be a helpful and healing experience for grieving children. Writing can be in the form of poetry, letter writing, journal writing, keeping a diary, essays, or reflections on a specific topic (e.g., write a letter telling your parent or loved one good-bye).

Children can use writing for stating things that often cannot be said aloud, and it can be beneficial in many ways:

- It can give the children a better understanding of happenings.
- It helps them formulate and clarify their thoughts.
- It helps to make feelings more clear and understandable.
- It relieves some of the frustrations and anger the child is feeling.
- It may help make the loss real and acceptable.
- It may help the child to put an ending to the story about the death.
- It enables the children to explore and express their hopes, fears, fantasies, and realities.

Writing can be a means of self-support; an outlet children can use when other social support is unavailable. It can provide them with a "fully accepting friend" at that moment. Also, once a child has recorded his or her memories on paper, he or she does not have to be preoccupied with thoughts of forgetting about that person.

Although writing during the grief process may be a valuable coping tool for some bereaved children, it may not be appropriate for all children or in all circumstances. Individual timing must be considered since at some points in the grief process exploration of painful emotions can lead to a greater sense of vulnerability and a decreased ability to cope with grief. Writing about the death may be very painful for the child, thus it should be an activity of choice. Also, some children express difficulty and frustration with the content or quality of their writing. They need to be given the option not to write and not to disclose their writings within a group unless they feel it to be in their best interest.

I also give the child the option to share his or her writings with me. If they choose to share, it is sometimes therapeutic for them to read it out loud. Below are some suggestions for topics that the children might write about:

- Write a letter to your parent about a problem you are having.
- Special memory that I have about you.
- What I miss the most about you.
- What I wish I'd said.
- What I wish I hadn't said.
- What I'd like to ask you.
- How I feel right now.
- Telling you good-bye.
- What I didn't like about you.
- What I dream about.
- Possible alternatives to a problem I am having.

They may want to write in a journal or diary about their own thoughts, feelings, and observations of the day.

Below is a poem written by four children whose mother died of cancer. The children are Vince, age 14; Brian, age 12; Jay, age 10; and Amy, age 8.

This may seem a little funny,
    But it's really true,
It's from your three big sonnies,
    And your little daughter, too!

You taught us how to think up rhymes,
    We wanted one to last,
We thank you for all the good times,
    We really had a blast!

We're a bunch of hams; we must confess,
    But you and Dad together created this mess.
Let's get serious now; we'll stop kidding around,
    We've got things to say; we need to cover some ground!

Dear Mom,

Thank you, Mom, for all you've done,
    Some games we've lost; some games we've won.
Thanks for singing and laughter and help from you,
    A home to be proud of and hard work, too!

For choosing a most special dad with grandparents
        Tried and true,
For super uncles, loving aunts, and a little Megan, too.
    But most of all, before we're through,
We want to thank God for giving us *you*!

We're your four little chicks as you can see,
    We love you so much, on that we agree!

I'm Vincent, your Teenager, I've loved you the longest,
    I'm Brian, your Wrestler, my love is the strongest.
I'm Jay, your Bird, my love you can't sever,
    I'm Amy, Miss Priss, I'll love you forever!

Music

Another tool that can be used with children is music. Music can be very powerful, yet gentle and nonthreatening to the child. Music can bring to the surface all those emotions that a child has been afraid to voice. It can encourage the child to let her barriers down and give her the freedom to cry or not to cry.

Certain songs can remind the child of earlier times in his life when he felt secure and felt unconditional love. In the privacy of his home, it may bring back memories of laughter and tears.

31

Music can be very calming and peaceful especially when it is used with a restless or hyperactive child. You will want to be careful of the selection because it can also be a stimulant. You might want to encourage parents to put on soothing music for the child to go to sleep by.

Music also helps some people to feel beautiful inside, feel more confident, and may encourage the child to see themselves as having self-worth again.

Storytelling

Another tool that I use with some children is to tell them a story, and let them fill in the blanks. Many of the words I leave blank are feeling words. I also let the child put an ending to the story. Storytelling provides a nonthreatening way to better understand the child's experiences and feelings and to look for major themes the child is verbally telling you. Exercise 24 is an example of a story I made up for a young boy whose pet and father had died.

Before the story, the boy would answer my questions, but would not expand on any subject. As he filled in the blanks of the story, he opened up and described how he felt about his losses.

5

USING ART

When working with children in grief, I use art because it offers a strong supportive basis for communication with the child. I find that children's feelings and thoughts (conscious and unconscious) flow freely onto the drawing paper.

A child's drawings express emotions and thoughts that can alert us to unmet needs or can assure us of the child's strengths and growth. Drawings can communicate unspoken wants, needs, and anxieties. The discoveries of these can help those in contact with the child to respond appropriately to meet these needs. Adults can then provide the support to lessen any fear or confusion that the child in grief may feel.

Furth (1981) says that it is most productive in studying pictures to begin with what is known and work toward the unknown. Reading a drawing requires paying careful attention to every detail, observing how everything is related or not related, and constantly searching for the possible significance of this data. Positioning, movement, colors, shapes, patterns, the number of objects, and how the picture corresponds to the real world are only a few of the aspects that must be critically examined before the impressions can be formulated to interpret the picture's meaning.

There are dangers involved in attempting to analyze children's drawings. It is quite difficult not to read into the picture what one already knows or suspects to be there, and the interpreter can project his own unconscious material into the person's drawing. It is a very serious undertaking to counsel an individual using as a tool the reflections from the person's unconscious realm. In order to analyze drawings properly, one must have the necessary professional training.

Since my professional training is limited in the area of interpreting children's drawings, I always encourage the child to tell me about their picture—what the picture is about, if there is a story taking place in the picture, how they felt when they drew it, how they feel now, etc. This not only encourages better understanding and communication between the child and me, but it also gives me a guide about what to observe for and sometimes what questions to ask the child.

In working with children and art, you will find yourself feeling for the child as he shares his drawings because these are an expression of that child's personality (his own self-portrait). The child is taking a chance on sharing his most inner feelings and life experiences. You must be willing to let the child share his emotions, hopes, pain, and expectations.

Symbols in drawings begin at the unconscious level. When an individual can be helped to bring into consciousness and assimilate what his symbolic language is trying to teach him, he can begin to work toward needed changes in his life. In the case of a child, the cooperation of certain adults may be needed to bring about the necessary change.

There are certain symbols that I do observe for in the drawings of children in grief:

1. Death is often represented by white skeletons, ghosts, monsters, poison signs, angels, or beings that have wings. The colors used are often white or black.
2. Hearts or birds may symbolize the soul.
3. Rain could represent purification and cleansing.
4. Purple can represent what is spiritual and perhaps even possessive or possessing.
5. Red is often used if there was a violent death.
6. Anger is represented by the colors red and black, by strong definite lines, or by the drawing of lightning.
7. No arms or legs give the impression of helplessness or perplexity.
8. Standing or sitting on some kind of base may mean that the child has a firm or solid support at home.
9. Crosshatching often signifies anxiety.
10. Windows in a home allow light to come in, make it possible for one to view outside, or may make it possible for one on the outside to see what is on the inside.
11. A home without windows may mean that the child does not want anyone to see into their home life.
12. Glass or clouds can symbolize the spirit (the child's spirit or God's).
13. Fire and smoke often indicate the need for love and warmth.
14. An individual who draws stick figures is often uncomfortable about revealing either to himself or to others his authentic self.
15. If the drawing is not clear because of so many lines, it often represents confusion. Also, when a child is confused as what to feel about their loss, they often draw a face that is without expression or "neutral."
16. Sadness can be represented by the color blue or by the drawing of rivers, raindrops, or clouds.
17. A heart with an arrow or a crack through it can represent a broken heart.

I have the children draw pictures in six different areas:[*]

1. How their face looks with different feelings.
2. How they see death.
3. Nightmares or dreams they have been having since their loved one died.
4. How they saw their family before the death, and how they see the family since the death.
5. How they see themselves now since the loss.
6. Some extemporaneous drawings.

Faces and Feelings

In having them draw how their face looks with different feelings, I want them to be aware of the many different feelings they can have and how their body reacts with these feelings.

Figure 1 is an example of how several of the children have drawn their sad faces. Notice the clouds hanging over the face and the tears. Often the face is colored blue or black. Some of the children do not draw tears with their sad faces.

Figure 2 was drawn by an angry seven-year-old boy whose father was killed in a

---

[*]See Appendix A for figures which illustrate drawings of children.

car accident. The figure on the left is the boy being mad at the lady who killed his dad. The head on the right is the lady who killed his dad. The boy said, "She is smiling because she is happy that she killed my daddy. She must have been happy because she had been drinking."

Death

In having them draw what death is, I can begin to understand what they have been told about the death and what level of understanding they have. Their drawings also give clues as to what is confusing for the child, what needs to be cleared up, and what fears or questions they have about death.

Figure 3 was drawn by a nine-year-old boy whose father died at home from a brain tumor. He described death and his drawing as a person going through a black tunnel. At the end of the tunnel is the light of heaven and around the tunnel are the "paws of fear."

Figure 4 was drawn by a seven-year-old boy whose father was killed in a truck accident. Death is the two purple monsters. The one on the left walks around on earth and snatches people. The one on the right is the "most dangerous" because he has wings and can fly around to snatch people. The boy said, "I am most scared of the one that flies because he could snatch me, but probably won't because I'm too strong." Notice how tall he drew himself to reach the clouds and sun. He stated, "I drew myself big so that I can reach Heaven and be with my dad," and smiles thinking about being with his dad.

Figure 5 was drawn by a ten-year-old boy after his mother died of cancer. Notice the soul (heart) traveling up the stairs to Heaven, then at the gates of Heaven, an angel carries the soul to enter Heaven. The boy has a very healthy concept of death.

Dreams and Nightmares

The children's drawings of dreams and nightmares usually reveals the many fears, guilt, and the confusion they are dealing with.

Figure 6 was drawn by a nine-year-old girl after her little brother died of leukemia. She dreamed that she was a small girl wandering around in the dark looking for her brother and not being able to find him. She is crying because she can't find her brother and is afraid that she will never see him again. See how overwhelming death is to children, and how small and helpless one feels in coping with it.

Family Before and After

I often have the child draw a picture of how they saw their family before the death and/or a picture of how they see their family after the death. These drawings often tell me about the changes going on in the family—how secure the child felt before the death and how secure he or she feels now, who is important in the child's life, the pain and problems the child may now be dealing with, etc. Also, sharing about their family gives the children a

35

chance to tell their story and a chance to begin to put an ending to their story about death. It gives them a foundation on which to rebuild their lives.

Figure 7 was drawn by a fourteen-year-old boy. He drew a picture of what his family was like before his mother died of cancer. From the drawing you can see the closeness of the family and that they did things together such as football games, movies, and making tacos.

How They See Themselves

I have the children draw how they see themselves at this time in their life. I listen and observe for clues to self-esteem, guilt, helplessness, strengths, and if the child has hope. I also tune into how the child sees himself physically and can occasionally pick up on a physical problem the child may be having. I then encourage the family to get the child to a medical doctor for a good check-up.

Figure 8 was drawn by a father of four children whose wife had died of cancer six months before this drawing. He described himself as the shepherd looking after his four baby sheep. This father was having to deal with his own grief, and at the same time was feeling overwhelmed with work and with trying to be both mother and father to the children. He felt like he was not meeting all of his children's needs. Notice how he is behind the sheep and not yet leading them, however, the drawing of the shepherd represents his love and concern for them. He is a fairly strict father, and I think this shows with the drawing of the staff.

Extemporaneous Drawings

Occasionally, I have the children draw extemporaneous pictures.

Figure 9 was drawn by a ten-year-old boy whose father died of a brain tumor, and this boy had this dream several times. He dreamed that he was staying at a friend's house playing when monsters came through the window. The boy picked up a bat to fight off the monsters while his friend hid and threw darts. This boy had been disappointed in how some of his friends and relatives had supported him during his father's illness and death; hence, the friend hiding. In the right-hand corner, dead mice came to life, stood up, and pointed at the monsters. The monsters then left. Notice how the dead mice came back to life in time to protect this boy as he wanted his father to. The games up in the air seem to represent the upheaval a child can feel after losing the security a father provides, and of the loss of a normal family routine. The monsters represent death and how frightening and fierce death can seem to a child.

36

6

HELPING YOUR CHILDREN WITH GRIEF

The first thing you can do is be human and share your grief with your child. Be able to cry with your child so you can then laugh with him or her when all is well again. Too often adults try to protect their children from hurt and pain by covering up their own grief, "I must be strong for my child so that they know I am in control." As difficult as it may be, the child has to deal with the death. You will find that if you are open about your own feelings, it gives your child permission to grieve.

It is not wrong to express your own emotions of grief whether it be to shed some tears or to say a word of anger or regret. Anger, tears, guilt, despair, and protest are natural reactions to family disorganization, and you need to reassure your child that their feelings are normal.

It is important to encourage your child to talk and to ask questions as often as he or she wants. A younger child may ask the same questions over and over, and it will take patience in answering these questions. It is not that the child isn't hearing you, but the child is trying to make sense out of the death. It is a healthy element in the grief process. Children need answers to put things about the death in sequence and to help them form a story in their own mind. This helps them work toward incorporating the reality of the loss.

Be open and honest in your answers and if you don't know an answer, it is alright to say, "I don't know but we will learn together." Do not tell your child what he or she will later need to unlearn, so avoid half-truths. Do not go into lengthy, complicated explanations about the death; simple direct answers are the best.

With some children you may need to provide a natural quiet time for them to open up. Putting a puzzle together or taking a walk may provide that time. Be careful not to push children into talking about it if they are not ready to deal with it. They have a right to freedom of expression and a right to their defenses. The parent can allow each child to experience the full range of feelings toward the deceased on the child's own timetable. Working through grief goes slowly, and we must not be in too big of a hurry to get ourselves and our child "back to normal."

When the child is ready to talk, that is the time to listen. If you ask the child to postpone their questions or feelings, you will block communications. What you are really saying to the child is that what he or she has to say is not important at that time. They may not be willing to share with you at a later time.

Be careful not to tell the child what to feel or for how long. Some parents tell their child that they will probably feel depressed for several months and then if that child has some happy moments, he or she often feels guilty because they aren't feeling depressed. Also, be careful not to criticize or seem shocked by the child's statements of feelings. If a child tells you that he is angry at the parent that has died, don't make him feel guilty for that anger. He probably is angry because the parent has left him, and he will work through that anger with your support.

Do not tell children how well they are doing if they are not grieving. They will then continue to delay their grief so that you will be proud of them (e.g., "My child is taking it so well; she never cries."). Also, telling children to "be brave" sounds as if you are minimizing their loss. Don't be afraid to cause tears. Crying is like a safety valve and is normal and helpful. The worst thing possible is for the child to repress crying. The child who keeps her grief bottled up inside may later find a release in a more serious explosion.

With children, what you do and how you do it is often more important than what you say. It is important to get physically close to sit and listen. It helps to hold or touch your children because they often need the warmth of an adult's body to calm and reassure them that they will be taken care of. Also, children become discouraged and lose emotional energy. Children can regain that energy when someone puts a loving arm around them, touches their hand, or pats them on the back.

If you are caught up in your own grief and feel that you cannot meet your child's needs, don't feel guilty about it. Sometimes this happens, and it is then helpful to find an adult friend or relative that can help provide emotional support to your child. You can also look for people to fill in other gaps left by a parent's death (e.g., getting a neighbor or someone at church to take the child on outings). As you work through your own grief, you will be more able to meet your child's needs. Make it clear to your child that someone will look out for him or her and reassure your child that there is enough money for food and toys.

After losing one parent, a child usually fears that their surviving parent may also die and won't be there to care for him or her. Never promise a child that you will not die; that is a promise you cannot keep. I have counseled some children that have lost both parents within a year's time. Point out to your child that your health is fine and that they will be taken care of. Try not to disrupt the child's daily routine anymore than you have to. If you have to leave a younger child, be reliable about returning at the expected time to pick him up. If you are to be late, call your child and explain that you will be late. Also, help your child to focus on the day's routine so that he can predict when to expect you. Assure him that you will be thinking of him while apart.

Try to avoid subsequent losses immediately after a major loss such as a change in schools, church, or neighborhoods. You don't want to cut off your child's ties with old friends or grandparents. Too many changes just add more stress to an already stressful situation. Also, too many changes may cause the child to delay his or her grief. Children often need to be around their loved one's possessions and environment to grieve.

Encourage the child to remember and talk about the person who has died. By sharing memories of that person, you reaffirm their worth and life. One should recall and speak freely of the "good things" and "not-so-good things" that the loved one did. Be realistic about your memories so that the child will not make the person larger than life-size in his memory. You might put a picture of the lost loved one in your child's room or make up a memory box that can hold the loved one's personal items (such as a pocket knife or a watch). This lets the grieving child know that his loved one will always be remembered. At the funeral home's viewing room, you might place a printed note on the table with blank pages of paper. The note could ask guests to write about a memory of the deceased so it can be shared with the children.

Do not be surprised if your children regress in their behavior. They may regress in one area such as whining or wetting the bed but not in all areas. It is common and usually does not become a long-term problem if you are supportive to them during their grief. You may need to leave a night light on or dig out a favorite toy or blanket that they had as a younger child. They also like snuggling against a warm, soft surface such as a blanket, and they may need extra clothing to feel warm and more secure. You might want to give your children special foods such as ones which remind them of earlier, easier times (e.g., soft foods such as puddings, mashed potatoes, or soups).

If your children are active a great deal of the time since their loss, try to provide some quiet time for them each day. This can be done by giving them a warm bath, rubbing their backs, listening to music, or teaching them relaxing exercises. You may want to put the radio on softly at night until they are asleep. Be alert for exhaustion in a hyperactive child.

It is not unusual for children to have some problems in school for several months after their loss. Be alert to a drop in grades, lack of attention, daydreaming, hostility, and withdrawal from friends. It is important to alert the child's teachers, principal, and counselor of the child's loss, and then work closely with them over the next several months in helping your child. You might even want to encourage the teacher to lighten the work load of the child for awhile. Grief takes a lot of energy, and there isn't much energy left to concentrate on doing tasks. You may need to give your child concrete suggestions on how to get his or her mind on tasks, how to tackle one problem at a time, or make lists for things the child needs to do. Also, it might help to have a set time to talk about the loss so that the child can spend the rest of her or his time concentrating on tasks.

Children in grief will be more prone to illnesses such as colds, flu, sore throats, ear infections, skin reactions, muscle tightness, burning on urination, and eating disorders. Be alert to your child's physical needs, and see a medical doctor if a problem arises. Encourage your children to eat balanced meals and to drink plenty of water. Try to keep them away from junk food, especially sugar and caffeine. See that they get plenty of exercise and rest. Even if they aren't sleeping well at night, try to set a routine for their bedtime. It is normal for them not to sleep well because of nightmares and fears.

Your child may have some anger, guilt and/or fears to deal with. Help your child to deal with his feelings in constructive ways such as working with play dough or clay; hammering nails; hitting a punching bag or pillow; walking, jogging, or playing a team sport; and use of music, art, or creative writing. Grief is energy so be creative with it.

You feel so bad about your child's loss that it is easy to be too permissive with the child, and you may end up spoiling the child. Most children in grief say that they need guidelines and discipline to know that their parent is still in control and is still able to care for them.

Encourage your child to ask for what he or she needs. For example, if she is having a "bad" day, she may need to ask for a hug or she may need to ask for help in getting organized.

Remember that the loss of a child is very difficult on the surviving siblings. Children say that the most difficult times came when they did not know what was occurring, so talk with your child. Also, be aware that siblings will have a mixture of emotions—sad that the relationship has ended, worried that the protection and care given by the death of the sibling is no longer available, and yet relieved that with the sibling's absence, she is now more of the center of attention in the family. Children will often feel guilty about these mixed emotions even if it is related to normal sibling rivalry.

Some children fear that they may have the same symptoms and will die at exactly the same age as their brother or sister. Also, the surviving child may feel severe separation anxiety and may be reluctant about going to school.

The parent's handling of the death and their own grief reactions will have a definite effect on young children. Some parents become over-protective, displaying favoritism or restrictiveness with the surviving children; some may resent the surviving child; some may attempt to recreate in that child some of the qualities of the deceased child; or some may unintentionally minimize contact with the surviving child because the living child may be a painful reminder of the child now lost.

It is easy to become overwhelmed by many demands and responsibilities that double after the death of a spouse. A parent usually moves closer to the children after a spouse's death, and their children often give them "a reason to go on living." Try not to become too dependent on your children to fill the role of your mate. A parent's dependence on the children can result in the family's failure to accomplish its developmental tasks. Also, the parent who turns to the older children for emotional and functional support may diminish his or her authority over them. The surviving parent must assume the child-rearing tasks, must be responsible for decision-making, and must assume some of the responsibilities of the deceased parent.

It takes time for family members to redefine their roles and to identify their new family unit. Just remember that you do not have to do things precisely the way your spouse would have wanted, and you cannot be both parents to your children. If you become overwhelmed by the many demands of parenting and homemaking, ask for help (e.g., a woman may need to find someone to keep the car in good condition, and a man may need to hire someone to clean house).

Getting through birthdays, special family days, and the holidays is difficult for a grieving family. It will never be quite the same. You may not be able to function at your usual level so take one day at a time, and be realistic about what you can handle. Recognize that you need to set limits, and do those things which are meaningful to your family. Reduce holiday pressures by eliminating or reassigning those activities that are not as important to you. Do not be afraid to make changes. This may be the time to start new family traditions while you hang on to those which help to alleviate some of the pain. Know that whatever you choose to do this year, you may decide to handle things differently next year.

Above all, remember that your situation is unique. What worked for someone else may not feel right for you. Trust yourself; if it makes the special days more bearable for you and your family, then do it. Remember many families discovered that when the "special day" arrives, it truly was not as bad as they had anticipated.

Let your children know that it will take time before they feel better and that healing will happen. Reassure them that it is going on even in their hurting and that hurting is part of the cure.

If necessary, get professional help for your child or the entire family. A few sessions at the time of crisis could prevent a child from developing long-term problems. Be aware of some of the danger signs that say your child may need help. Some danger signs are isolating himself, showing a great amount of anger by smashing things or slamming doors, giving away possessions and mentioning suicide, problems in school, using alcohol or drugs, physical problems such as a large loss or gain of weight, etc. It is helpful to look at your situation realistically and to trust your instincts. You can usually tell when your child is getting into trouble. Remember that many children have only one parent, and children from single-parent homes can do well in life. Above all, just *love* and *listen* to your child.

APPENDIX A
Children's Art

FIGURE 1: *Sad Faces*

FIGURE 2: *A Boy's Anger (following his father's death)*

FIGURE 3: *Depiction of Father's Death*

FIGURE 4: *A Boy's Fear (death is depicted as monstrous)*

FIGURE 5: *A Positive Image of Death*

FIGURE 6: *Death as an Overwhelming Event*

FIGURE 7: *Family Closeness before Death Occurred*

FIGURE 8: *Father's Feeling after Death of His Spouse*

FIGURE 9: *Depiction of Fight with Death*

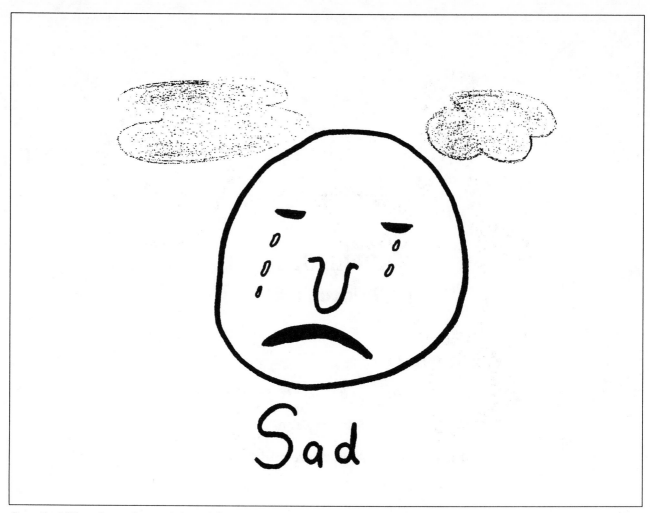

Several children have drawn their sad faces. Notice the clouds hanging over the face and the tears. Often the face is colored blue or black. Some children do not draw tears with their sad faces.

FIGURE 1

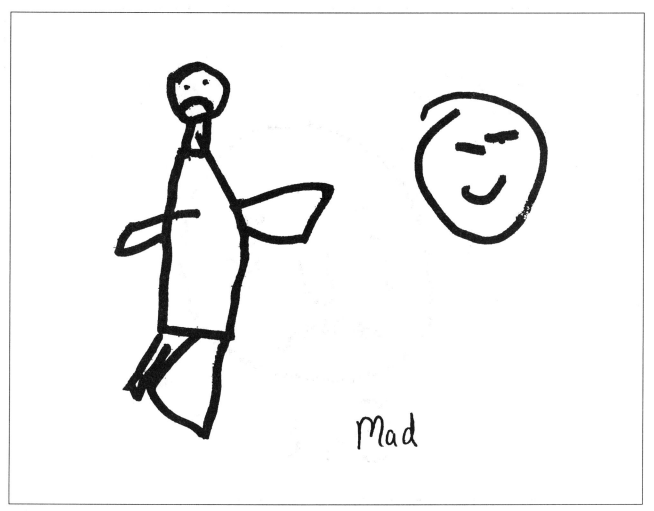

Drawing by an angry seven-year-old boy whose father was killed in a car accident. The figure on the left is the boy being mad at the lady who killed his dad. The head on the right is the lady who killed his dad. The boy said, "She is smiling because she is happy that she killed my daddy. She must have been happy because she had been drinking."

FIGURE 2

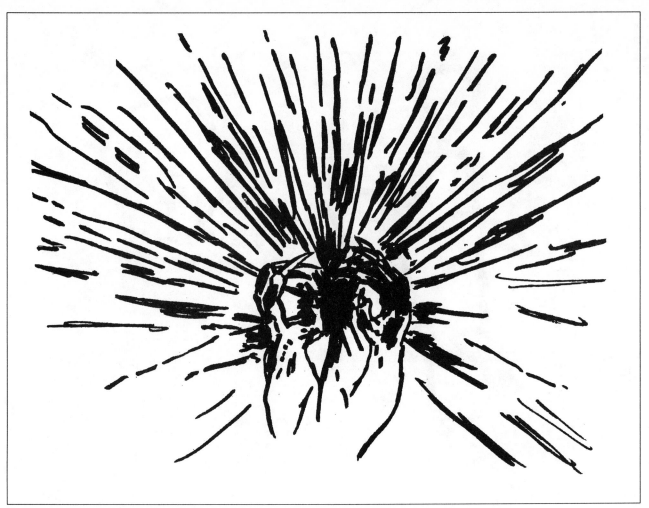

Drawing by a nine-year-old boy whose father died at home from a brain tumor. He described death and his drawing as a person going through a black tunnel. At the end of the tunnel is the light of heaven and around the tunnel are the "paws of fear."

FIGURE 3

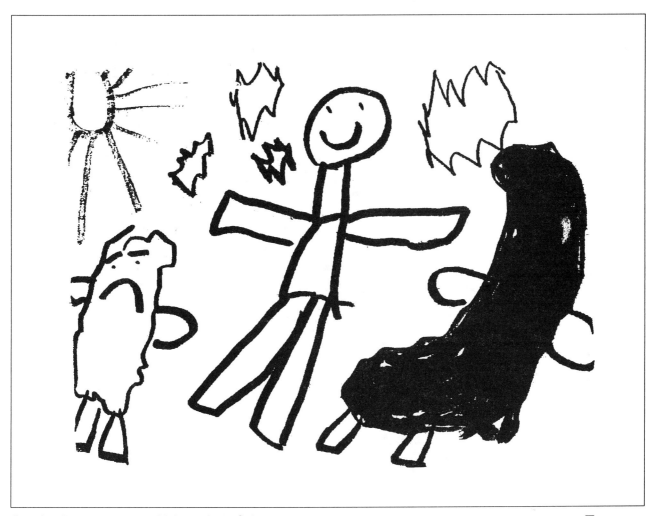

Drawing by a seven-year-old boy whose father was father was killed in a truck accident. Death is the two purple monsters. The one on the left walks around on earth and snatches people. The one on the right is the "most dangerous" because he has wings and can fly around to snatch people. The boy said, "I am most scared of the one that flies, because he could snatch me, but probably won't because I'm too strong." Notice how tall he drew himself to reach the clouds and sun. He stated, "I drew myself big so that I can reach heaven and be with my dad," and smiles thinking about being with his dad.

FIGURE 4

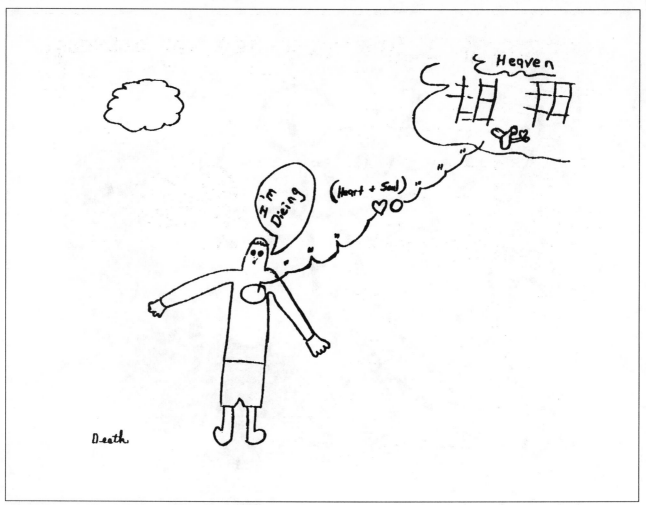

Drawing by a ten-year-old boy after his mother died of cancer. Notice the soul (heart) traveling up the stairs to Heaven, then at the gates of Heaven, an angel carries the soul to enter Heaven. The boy has a very healthy concept of death.

FIGURE 5

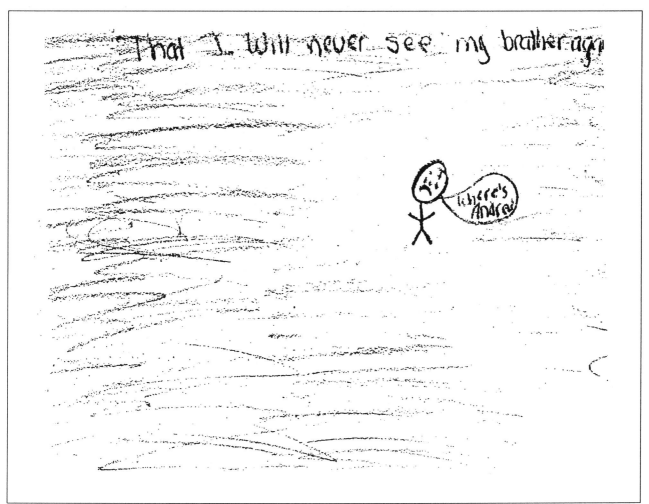

Drawing by a nine-year-old girl after her little brother died of leukemia. She dreamed that she was a small girl wandering in the dark looking for him but not being able to find him. She is crying because she can't find him and is afraid she will never see him again. Note how overwhelming death is to children, and how small and helpless one feels in coping with it.

FIGURE 6

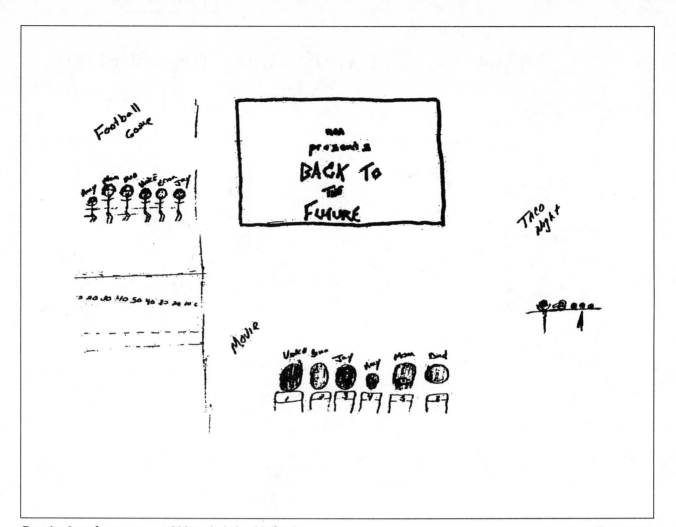

Drawing by a fourteen-year-old boy depicting his family before his mother died of cancer. Note their closeness and they did things together—football games, movies, and making tacos.

FIGURE 7

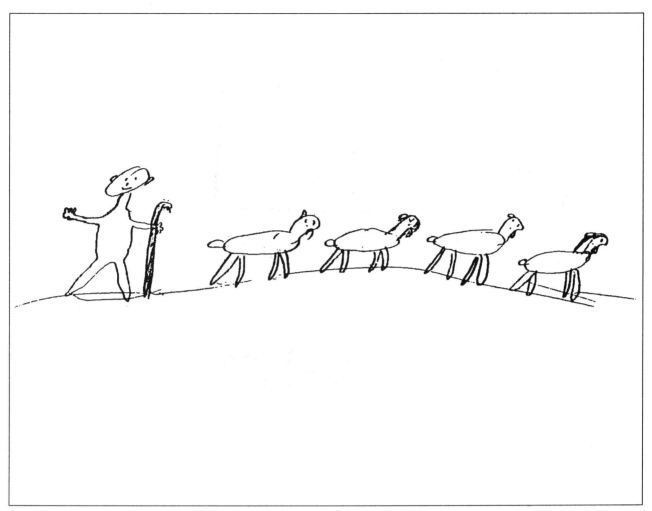

Drawing by a father of four whose wife had died of cancer six months earlier. This father was feeling overwhelmed with work and with trying to be both mother and father to the children. He felt that he was not meeting all of this children's needs; notice how he is behind the sheep and not yet leading them.

FIGURE 8

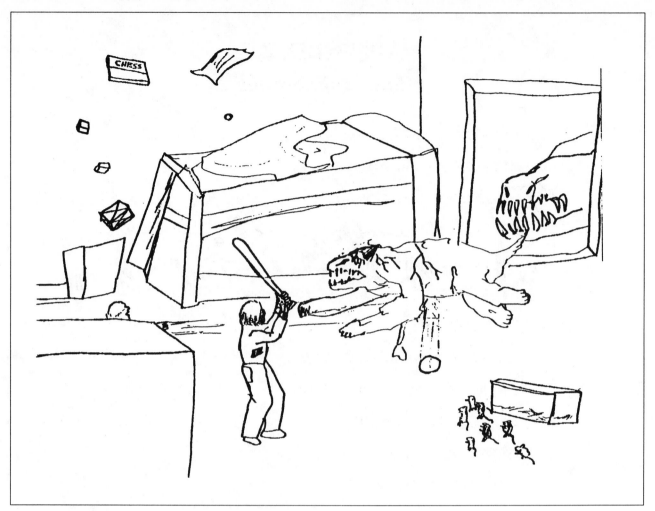

Drawing of a dream image by a ten-year-old boy whose father died of a brain tumor. He dreamed he was at a friend's house playing when monsters came through the window. The monsters represent death and how frightening and fierce death can seem.

FIGURE 9

APPENDIX B
Handout Exercises

Find Someone Who. . .

Has seen the Atlantic Ocean (East).	Has camped outside in a tent.	Can speak another language besides English.	Plays the Piano.
Can snow ski.	Has flown in an airplane.	Likes to sing.	Has had a speaking part in a play.
Has written a poem.	Plays baseball or softball.	Makes their bed every morning.	Can make their own meal to eat.

Feeling Good

Exercise 2

Some people make us feel good. List the ways these people make you feel good about who you are and what you do:

1. My teacher makes me feel good when she (he) _____

_____

_____

2. My friends make me feel good when they _____

_____

_____

3. My parent(s) makes me feel good when he (she) _____

_____

_____

4. I make myself feel good when I _____

_____

_____

5. I make other people feel good when I _____

_____

_____

Grief Reactions

Listed below are some grief feelings or reactions you might have had. First, check in the left-hand column the reactions you have had. Then, in the right-hand column, check if you think it is "OK" or "Not OK" to have these reactions.

Reactions I Have Had		OK To Have	Not OK To Have
☐	1. Tears	☐	☐
☐	2. Restlessness (hard time sitting still)	☐	☐
☐	3. Low level of energy	☐	☐
☐	4. Loneliness	☐	☐
☐	5. Relieved that the death is over	☐	☐
☐	6. Wondering who will take care of me now	☐	☐
☐	7. Find it hard to concentrate	☐	☐
☐	8. Find it hard to care about things going on around me	☐	☐
☐	9. Anger at God	☐	☐
☐	10. Anger at loved one for dying	☐	☐
☐	11. Nightmares/Dreams	☐	☐
☐	12. Fear that I might die the same way my loved one did	☐	☐
☐	13. Guilt or regrets that I sometimes got mad at my loved one when he or she was alive	☐	☐

Changes

Complete each statement:

1. If I could change how I look, I would _____
   _____

2. If I could change my grades, I would _____
   _____

3. If I could change my family, I would _____
   _____

4. If I could change my home, I would _____
   _____

5. If I could change my mother/father, I would _____
   _____

6. If I could change the world, I would _____
   _____

7. If I could change a bad habit, I would _____
   _____

8. If I could change my teacher, I would _____
   _____

9. If I could change my talents, I would _____
   _____

10. If I could change my friends, I would _____
    _____

Grief

True or False

Check the appropriate boxes if you think the following statements are *true* or *false*.

		TRUE	FALSE
1.	People die because they have been "bad" .... ☐		☐
2.	It is OK to cry .... ☐		☐
3.	There are some things about death that I don't understand .... ☐		☐
4.	I must be strong for those around me .... ☐		☐
5.	People that get mad at God will be punished .... ☐		☐
6.	I fear that I may die of the same disease/accident my loved one did .... ☐		☐
7.	I did not always love my parent or sibling that died .... ☐		☐
8.	If I had been nicer to my loved one, she or he wouldn't have died .... ☐		☐
9.	I wish I would have told my loved one something before he or she died .... ☐		☐
10.	My dead loved one was always good .... ☐		☐
11.	I wish my living loved one would have been the one to die .... ☐		☐
12.	Pain is part of the healing process .... ☐		☐

Constructive Ways of Dealing
With Your Feelings

1. Fears

   We all have fears sometimes. It helps to find someone you can trust to talk to about these fears. Identify what you are afraid of and call it by name. It may help to write these fears down or draw a picture of them. If the fears happen more at night, you may want to have a night light on.

2. Anger

   If you are angry, you can choose to deal with it by getting it out or you can choose to continue to be angry. Anger is energy, and you can choose to use that energy in creative ways, such as:

   a. Art–take a paint brush or crayon, and color your feelings.

   b. Music–listening to or creating music.

   c. Writing—you may want to put your feelings into words in a journal, writing poetry, a short story, or reflections (e.g. "How I feel right now.").

   d. Physical Release—anger can be released by hitting a pillow or punching bag, by hammering on some nails, jogging, working with clay, or playing a physical game such as tennis, basketball, or racquetball. You may even want to yell in private while you are playing some games or while taking a shower.

   e. Relaxing Exercises–you may want to try a relaxing exercise.

3. Guilt or Regrets

   You may find yourself saying "if only..." Sometimes we carry guilt around inside of us, and it makes us feel like we are all tied up in knots. You may need to identify your guilt and admit it belongs to you. You may need to ask yourself, "What does it take to forgive myself?" Remember that guilt is not a "bad" or "good" feeling, but rather that we feel as we feel.

Support

Check which influence each person(s) has on you:

	Helper	Hinderer	No Influence
1. Parent			
2. Friend (name)			
3. Teacher			
4. Grandparents			
5. Neighbor			
6. Sunday School Teacher			
7. Counselor			
8. Principal			
9. Coach			
10. Pastor/Priest			
11. Brother/Sister			

I Believe in My Abilities

1. I believe I that I am _____

   _____

2. I believe that I can _____

   _____

3. I believe that people like me because _____

   _____

4. I believe that I am kind to _____

   _____

5. I believe that I am a good listener when _____

   _____

6. I believe that I have the talent of _____

   _____

7. I believe that I could _____

   _____

Taking Care of Yourself

1. Nutrition

    It is easy for children in grief to eat a lot of "junk" food. You may want to eat all of the time (trying to fill up the empty feeling), or you may have a loss of appetite. It is important to eat daily portions of food from each of the four basic food groups (meat, milk, fruit/vegetable, bread/cereal). Let's also discuss what good snacks might be (yogurt, cheese, apple, raisins, nuts, carrots, etc.).

2. Daily Exercise

    Exercise is important so that your muscles can provide the appropriate pumping functions for nourishing and cleansing the body. Regular exercise is also the most effective means for controlling depression ("the blues"). Those chemicals of the brain which cause feelings of alertness and happiness are stimulated in exercise. Also, exercise will help you sleep better.

3. Drink Plenty of Water

    Under stress such as grief, the body muscles tighten up and use more body fluid. Water helps to maintain proper muscle tone by giving muscles their natural ability to contract and by preventing dehydration. Water also helps rid the body of waste. Adequate fluids depend on body weight (6 to 8 glasses a day). Pop and tea are not good because of the caffeine.

4. Rest and Relaxation

    It is important that regular rituals for rest are followed. Grief is an exhausting process emotionally. You need to replenish yourself. Physically you will be more prone to colds, sore throats, and the flu. It is important that your body has time to rest and regain its strength and energy. When you find yourself under stress or unable to slow down because you are too active, you may need to do some relaxation exercises. (Show them some deep breathing exercises or how to relax their muscles.)

5. Support You Have

    Find that person or persons who can give you support, and it may need to be outside the family. Someone that will listen to you without judging, will let you talk about your dead loved one or about a problem you may be having, and someone who will keep in confidence what you have said.

6. Learn to Ask for What You Need

    Sometimes you may have needs that others won't be able to see or understand, so it is important for you to learn how to ask for those needs to be met. You may need to ask for someone to listen to you, for a hug when you are hurting, or for your parent and/or teacher to help you with school work and with concentration. Don't assume that those around you know what you are thinking or feeling; you may have to tell them. Let's practice saying, "I need a hug."

7. Tears

Tears are a natural part of grief, and they help relieve stress. You must give yourself permission to cry. This is part of being human. Suppressing your tears may even be physically harmful because of the toxic substance some tears give off.

8. Laugh

Don't be afraid to laugh. It's healthy and is often needed to relieve tension. Laughter is the sunshine of the soul. You may even want to go to a movie that will make you laugh. Don't feel guilty about laughing. Just because you laugh doesn't mean that you aren't grieving or missing your loved one.

9. Remember:

a. Feel the pain; accept your emotions. They are part of grief. The pain is part of the healing process.
b. Death ends a life but it does not end a relationship. Memories go on in the survivor's mind. Let your loved one be with you by remembering.
c. You may not be grieving like those around you. What is grief to you may not be grief to someone else. It is all right because everyone grieves differently. Allow yourself to grieve your own way.
d. Allow yourself to accept the expressions of caring from others.
e. Escape for awhile and find a spot of peace and quiet.
f. Take days and things one at a time.
g. Give yourself a pat on the back for the things you do well, but don't try to be perfect.

Problem Solving

Answer each question below by circling the answer(s) which is most like what you think you would do if these situations would happen to you.

1. Someone laughs at you because you only have one parent.
   Do you:

   (a) Get mad and tell them it is none of their business.

   (b) Ignore them by walking away.

   (c) Keep the hurt inside for several days.

   (d) Explain briefly that your parent died.

   (e) Other _____

2. You wake up in the middle of the night because of a nightmare. Do you:

   (a) Hide your head and quietly cry to yourself.

   (b) Call out for your parent, and share your fears with that parent.

   (c) Keep quiet but lay awake for a long time afraid to go back to sleep.

   (d) Other _____

3. You worry that you might die of the same disease or accident your parent died of. Do you:

   (a) Share this fear with a family member or a friend.

   (b) Ask a professional nurse or doctor about the possibility.

   (c) Keep the worry to yourself so as not to upset anyone or have someone laugh at you.

   (d) Other _____

4. You are angry that your loved one has died. Do you:

   (a) Yell at members of your family.

   (b) Slam doors.

   (c) Take a walk or hit your pillow.

   (d) Feel guilty about your anger.

   (e) Other _____

Letter

Write a letter to your parent about a problem you are having:

Dear _____,

_____

_____

_____

_____

_____

_____

_____

_____

_____

_____

_____

_____

_____

_____

_____

_____

_____

Child of the Year

You have just been selected as "Child of the Year." Write what you think you did to deserve the award.

_____

_____

_____

_____

_____

_____

_____

_____

_____

_____

_____

_____

_____

_____

_____

_____

Evaluation

1. At first, I (did, did not) want to join this group because:

    _____

    _____

    _____

2. What did you like most about this group?

    _____

    _____

    _____

3. What did you like least about this group?

    _____

    _____

    _____

4. Should every child in grief join a support group like this one? _____

    Why? _____

    _____

    _____

5. If I could change something about this group, I would change:

    _____

    _____

    _____

Feelings

Describe times when you feel like this by completing these sentences:

1. I am embarrassed when _____

    _____

2. I am proud when _____

    _____

3. I am sad when _____

    _____

4. I am happiest when _____

    _____

5. I am scared when _____

    _____

6. I have the most fun when _____

    _____

7. I am lonely when _____

    _____

8. I cry when _____

    _____

9. I get mad when _____

    _____

Feelings

Mark the feeling or feelings you have when these things happen to you:

		Makes Me Feel Happy	Makes Me Feel Sad	Makes Me Feel Angry	Makes Me Feel Afraid
1	Getting praise on something I do.				
2.	Getting punished for something I did not do.				
3.	Doing my best.				
4.	Someone breaks a promise to me.				
5.	Having friends.				
6.	Seeing my mother/father cry.				
7.	Getting a "C" on my report card.				
8.	Doing something for my mother/father.				
9.	Remembering my dead loved one.				
10.	Keeping a secret.				
11.	Having a nightmare.				
12.	Losing someone I love.				

Getting to Know You

Write a word in each of the boxes that describes you, then on the lines tell why it describes you.

Getting to Know You

In each square, list the things you like to do by yourself:

In each square, list the things you like to do with others:

Strengths and Weaknesses

1. List two things that you like to do in your free time:

   A. _____

   B _____

2. List two strengths that you have:

   A _____

   B. _____

3. List a weakness that you have: _____

   _____

4. Name one person you would most want to be like: _____

   _____

5. My favorite food is: _____

6. What do you usually do when you are lonely? _____

   _____

7. What do you usually do when you are angry? _____

   _____

8. I am happiest when _____

9. The chore I like least to perform is _____

10. The school subject I like most is _____

11. I need to practice _____

12. Something that makes me laugh is _____

13. The best time of my day is _____

14. My most memorable moment is _____

15. I think that I am a good person because _____

   _____

Problem Solving

1. What do you usually do when you are angry? _____

   _____

   What other things could you do? _____

   _____

2. What do you usually do when you are anxious or nervous? _____

   _____

   What other things could you do? _____

   _____

3. What do you usually do when you are sad? _____

   _____

   What other things could you do? _____

   _____

4. What do you usually do when you miss your loved one that has died? _____

   _____

   What other things could you do? _____

   _____

5. What do you usually do when you are scared or afraid? _____

   _____

   What other things could you do? _____

   _____

Problem Solving

Write how you might feel and your best solution for each situation:

1. Situation—Your puppy has run away.

    Your Feelings: _____

    Your Solution: _____

2. Situation—You see your best friend cheating on a test.

    Your Feelings: _____

    Your Solution: _____

3. Situation—Your parent won't let you stay over at a friend's house for the night because you didn't do your household duties for the week.

    Your Feelings: _____

    Your Solution: _____

4. Situation—You are the only one of your friends that has just one parent, and you don't have rides to ball practice.

    Your Feelings: _____

    Your Solution: _____

5. Situation—You want to buy a new bike but you know your parent is short on money.

    Your Feelings: _____

    Your Solution: _____

6. Situation—Your friend wants you to fool around but you told your parent that you would go right home after school.

    Your Feelings: _____

    Your Solution: _____

Relationships

Use words to describe some of the people in your life:

1. My favorite person is _____

    because _____

2. My friend is _____

    because _____

3. My parent is _____

    because _____

4. My teacher is _____

    because _____

5. My grandparents are _____

    because _____

"Support I Have"

List four people you could talk to about any problem you were having, and check the appropriate box:

	Most of the Time	Some of the Time	Seldom
1. _____	☐	☐	☐
2. _____	☐	☐	☐
3. _____	☐	☐	☐
4. _____	☐	☐	☐

Remembering

Write a "memorable moment" in your life that you shared with your loved one that has died. Briefly describe why each was memorable.

1. Memorable Holiday _____

    _____

    _____

2. Memorable Trip _____

    _____

    _____

3. Memorable Party _____

    _____

    _____

4. Memorable Playtime _____

    _____

    _____

5. Memorable Meal _____

    _____

    _____

6. Memorable Achievements _____

    _____

    _____

A Day in the Life of Mark

Mark woke up on a bright, sunny day. It was Friday and as he jumped out of bed he said to himself, "I feel _____." Mark got dressed and went to the table to eat his favorite breakfast of _____. While eating, he talked to his mom about _____ then he left for school thinking about _____. At school, Mark saw his best friend _____ and felt _____.

They went to their classroom and as Mark saw his teacher he thought _____. They first took out their reading books and read. Reading was then followed by Mark's favorite subject _____. At ten o'clock the bell rang for recess, and Mark felt _____.

After recess Mark took a spelling test and got an "A" on it which made him feel _____. After lunch was math time. The teacher was explaining something new. Mark didn't understand it, and he felt _____ so he _____.

On the way home from school, Mark and _____ had fun kicking rocks and talking. Mark felt _____. When he got home, his mother asked him to feed his dog, Patches. Mark got the dog food from the kitchen and went to the back yard to feed Patches, but Patches was gone; someone had left the gate open. Mark felt _____ because _____.

Mark looked for Patches but couldn't find him. When Mark's dad got home from work, he helped Mark look for his dog and that made Mark feel _____. They looked everywhere in the neighborhood, and they stopped at several houses to ask if anyone had seen Patches, but no Patches. It was getting dark so Mark's dad said they had to give up looking. Mark felt _____, and he _____. Patches was his very best friend. They had fun running and playing ball together. He could tell Patches anything, and Patches would go on loving him.

That night Mark had a long face and was very quiet. His dad said, "I know this is a sad time for you, Mark, but don't give up yet. We will put an ad in the paper offering a reward and maybe someone has found Patches and will return him."

Put an ending to the story (do you think Mark got Patches back?)

APPENDIX C
References

Beckmann, R. *I'm Glad to Be Me*. Wichita: Self-Published, 1986.

Edwards, D. *Music Therapy and Grief*. Speech presented at a Growth Associates Seminar, Wichita, Kansas, October, 1984.

Fox, S. *Children's Anniversary Reactions to the Death of a Family Member*. Omega, 1984-85, Vol. 15, No. 4, pp. 291-305.

Furth, G. The Use of Drawings Made at Significant Times in One's Life. In Kubler-Ross, E. *Living With Death and Dying*. New York: Macmillan Publishing Co., 1981.

Grollman, E. *Explaining Death to Children*. Presentation at the American School Health Association Annual Convention, October, 1976.

Jewett, C. *Helping Children Cope With Separation and Loss*. Massachusetts: The Harvard Common Press, 1982.

Rosen, H. *Prohibitions Against Mourning in Childhood Sibling Loss*. Omega, 1984-85, Vol. 15, No. 4, pp. 307-316.

Williams, M. *The Velveteen Rabbit (2nd ed.)*. New York: Avon Books, 1982.

APPENDIX D
Books for Children

Abbott, S. *Old Dog*. New York: Coward, McCann and Geoghegen, 1972. (A story of a boy's first encounter with death and of his love for an old dog who will no longer share his life.)

Bartoli, J. *Nonna*. Irvington Hudson, N.Y.: Harvey House, 1975. (Nonna is dead but her family laughs as well as cries when they remember her, and her grandchildren treasure their memories of her.)

Bawden, N. *Squib*. Phila.: J. B. Lippincott Co., 1971. (Twelve-year-old Kate has difficulty accepting the drowning deaths of both her father and brother.)

Borack, B. *Someone Small*. New York: Harper & Row, 1969. (A gentle story of a little girl growing up, her younger sister, and a pet bird that dies).

Brenner, B. *Year in the Life of Rosie Bernard*. New York: Harper & Row, 1971. (For fifth- and sixth-grade children about responses to the death of a mother.)

Brooks, J. *Uncle Mike's Boy*. New York: Harper & Row, 1973. (How an eleven-year-old boy faces the death of a sister.)

Carrick, C. *Accident*. New York: Seabury Press, 1976. (Christopher's dog is killed by a pickup truck while they are walking together. The book deals honestly with the boy's feelings of guilt and anger, grief and tears, as he prepares to bury his dog.)

Cleaver, V. and Cleaver, B. *Grover*. New York: New American Library, 1975. (Grover's confusion is compounded because Grover knew his ailing mother killed herself with a gun although people said it was an accident.)

Conley, B. *Butterflies, Grandpa, and Me*. Springfield, Il.: Human Services Press, 1976. (Through the eyes of Richie, the reader learns about his very special relationship with his grandpa and his very special feelings when his grandpa dies.)

De Paola, T. *Nana Upstairs and Nana Downstairs*. New ed. New York: G. P. Putnam's Sons, 1973. (A sensitive picture book about a young boy's warm relationship with his grandmother and great-grandmother. After the great-grandmother dies, the boy begins to realize that death comes to everyone.)

Dobrin, A. *Scat*. New York: Scholastic Book Services, 1971. (Tells of a boy who likes jazz, a form of music his grandma calls "trash music." When the grandma dies, Scat chooses to say good-bye to her with his music.).

Fassler, J. *My Grandpa Died Today*. New York: Human Science Press, 1971. (About the love shared by a young boy and his grandfather. When grandpa dies, David as well as the adults cried. David also learns that Grandpa had not been afraid to die.)

Grollman, E. A. *Talking About Death: A Dialogue Between Parent and Child*. Boston: Beacon Press, 1976. (A paperback written as a sharing resource between adult and child. The death of a grandfather is used to discuss the reality factors and feelings associated with death.)

Johnson, J. and Johnson, M. *Tell Me, Papa*. Springfield, Il.: Human Services Press, 1978. (Explains death in simple, nonthreatening terms easily understood by children up to age ten.)

Johnson, J. and Johnson, M. *Where's Jess*? Springfield, Il.: Human Services Press, 1982. (For children who have lost a sister or brother. When her ten-month-old sister died suddenly, Heather (age two) needed desperately to know what happened.)

Klein, N. *Confessions of an Only Child*. New York: Pantheon Books, 1974. (Nine-year-old Antonia has ambivalent feelings about sharing her parents with a new baby, but when the baby dies at birth she feels sad.)

Krauss, R. *Growing Story*. New York: Harper & Row, 1947. (A picture story of the way things in nature grow and change just as a little boy grows.)

Lee, V. *The Magic Moth*. New York: Seabury Press, 1972. (Six-year-old Mark-O becomes wiser about death when his ten-year-old sister dies after a long illness.)

Levy, E. *Children Are Not Paper Dolls*. Springfield, Il.: Human Services Press, 1982. (This book is directed mainly to sibling bereavement.)

Miles, M. *Annie and the Old One*. Boston: Little, Brown and Company, 1971. (About a Navajo girl who cannot imagine her world without her grandmother. Annie delays learning to weave from Grandmother because she falsely believes this will keep Grandmother with her forever).

Rock, G. *The House Without a Christmas Tree*. New York: Alfred A. Knopf, 1974. (Deals with the death of a parent).

Sanford, D. *It Must Hurt Alot*. Portland, Oregon: Multnomah Press, 1986. (About feelings that occur when a younger child experiences loss.)

Shecter, B. *Someplace Else*. New York: Harper & Row, 1971. (Deals with the death of the father.)

Shortwell, L. R. *Adam Bookout*. New York: Viking Press, 1967. (An eleven-year-old discovers that running away does not solve his problems after his parents' fatal plane crash).

Stein, S. B. *About Dying An Open Book for Parents and Children Together*. New York: Walker and Co., 1974. (Assists adults in helping children understand death without using story characters).

Books for Adults

Bayly, J. *The Last Thing We Talk About.* Il.: Cook Publishing House, 1973.

Conley, B. *Handling the Holidays.* Il.: Creative Marketing, 1979.

Davidson, G. *Understanding Mourning.* Minneapolis: Augsbury Publishing House, 1984.

Dodd, R. *Helping Children Cope With Death.* Pennsylvania: Herald Press, 1984.

Dodd, R. *When Someone You Love Dies; An Explanation of Death for Children.* Tennessee: Abingdon Press, 1987.

Grollman, E. *Explaining Death to Children.* Boston: Beacon Press, 1967.

Heavilin, M. *Roses in December.* California: Here's Life Publishers, 1986.

Krementz, J. *How It Feels When a Parent Dies.* New York: Alfred A. Knopf, 1988.

Kubler-Ross, E. *On Children and Death.* New York: Macmillan Publishing Co., 1983.

Landorf, J. *Mourning Song.* New Jersey: Fleming H. Revell Company, 1974.

Manning, D. *Don't Take My Grief Away From Me.* Texas: In-Sight Books, Inc., 1979.

Patterson, L. & Sheldon, E. *The Counseling Process.* Boston: Houghton Mifflin Company, 1983.

Swindoll, C. *For Those Who Hurt.* Oregon: Multnomah Press, 1977.

Worden, W. *Grief Counseling and Grief Therapy.* New York: Springer Publishing Co., Inc., 1982.

Child Abuse and Neglect

A Guidebook for Educators and Community Leaders

Alan W. McEvoy and Edsel L. Erickson

THE EPIDEMIC OF CHILD ABUSE at home reaches into every school district and into thousands of classrooms. There, educators wrestle with the dilemmas over ethics and policy. How to respond?

Child Abuse and Neglect maintains that educators have become crucial front line troops in detecting and confronting abuse incidents. Schools, say the authors, serve communities ideally in this regard; yet their roles can be strengthened even more by better teacher training and understanding of key concepts—the central purpose of *Child Abuse and Neglect*.

Teachers will acquire better information on such matters as abuse definition; diagnosis; understanding high-risk students and families; and how youth welfare agencies operate—an insight that minimizes case frustration. Schools can become even more instrumental in the prevention and reduction of abuse through the use of several new curricula this book recommends.

Child Abuse and Neglect gives a ground-breaking treatment of the issues. Since its publication, the subject has sustained national attention. Such prominence now compounds an earlier problem with new ones: high-visibility media reports; pressure for action from school boards and agencies; government scrutiny of programs; and civil liability suits.

Even in this the intensified atmosphere, *Child Abuse and Neglect* remains one of the few books addressing the roles of schools and educators explicitly. More than ever this volume is indispensable.

CONTENTS: Involving schools ● Clarifying educators' roles ● Understanding abuse ● Identifying maltreatment ● Incest: a special case of exploitation ● Developing school policies ● Helping children and parents ● Programming for teenage parents ● Appendices, Bibliography, Index.

Cat. #525, ISBN 1-55691-052-5 .... $19.95

Children of Alcoholics

A Guide for Parents, Educators and Therapists (2nd Edition)
How to Help and Find Help for Children Trapped in Alcoholic Families

by Robert J. Ackerman, Ph. D.
Co-founder, National Association for Children of Alcoholics

IN THE FAMILY TROUBLED BY ALCOHOLISM, every member is affected; but the most seriously hurt are the children. Robert J. Ackerman, Ph. D. is a leader in the field of alcoholism and the family. In *Children of Alcoholics* he brings the wealth of many years in research and counseling to those charged with responsibility for the young.

Detailed yet non-technical, practical yet rich in insights, *Children of Alcoholics* is a ground-breaking book in the field of personality development and behavior. Ackerman carefully explains how the alcoholic family functions by compensation and accommodation, under the overriding theme of enabling alcohol consumption. On a positive note, he tells how a family can become more self-aware of its distorted coping strategies; how the effects of alcoholism upon the children can be minimized; and most important, how children from such families can succeed in life.

*"Bob Ackerman's book **Children of Alcoholics** is must reading for anyone involved in the well-being of children. His knowledge of the subject and leadership in the COA field are well-known."*

Janet Geringer Woititz, Ed.D.
Author of Adult Children of Alcoholics

"Dr. Ackerman's combination of information and resources makes his book an important reference for parents, educators and all helping professionals concerned about children of alcoholics."

Sharon Wegscheider-Cruse
Founding Board Chairperson of the
National Association for Children of Alcoholics

CONTENTS: The COA's world ● Development and personality among COAs ● School and teacher roles ● Administrator roles ● Suggestions for therapists and parents ● Recommendations for concerned parents ● Implications for therapy ● Resource materials ● Resource agencies ● References, Index

Cat. #277, ISBN 0671-64527-7 .... $7.95

Helping Obese Children

Weight Control Groups that Really Work!

by Roselyn Marin

LITTLE PROFESSIONAL ATTENTION has been given to childhood obesity; still less is said on what can be done to correct it. *Helping Obese Children* is a practical workbook meeting that need with a program structured for use where it will most likely succeed: in the school setting.

Author Roselyn Marin, a long-time school guidance counselor, developed her plan for *Helping Obese Children* in the best possible "laboratory" — her own elementary school. Here it quickly received the praise and approval of faculty, principal, students and parents.

Beginning with the concept of a special curriculum and social group—The Winners Club—Marin's program came to incorporate the whole range of personal development areas: self-image, nutrition information, food preparation, self-esteem, acceptance, peer group positive support, recreation, learning, motivational development, humor, games and fun. The Winners Club became the most popular group in her school's entire guidance program. What began as a twelve-week course became a year-round program with a waiting list of would-be members. Besides such popularity, objective success measurements were impressive.

Contents: Overview of obesity, causes, remedies • Getting started • Group orientation • 23 lessons and activities • "Why Am I Fat?" • Burning off calories • Balanced meals • The 4 food groups • Cholesterol • "Putting up" and "putting down" • Dressing slim • Cooking skills • Anorexia • Vegetables for health and weight control • Sugar and salt • Quizzes, final test, progress records, participation certificate, handout sheets

Cat. #495, ISBN 1-55691-049-5,
Softcover..$19.95

Ordering: See page 81

Our Secret Feelings

Activities for Children of Alcoholics in Support Groups

by Deborah Sharp Molchan

THIRTY-ONE MILLION American children have an alcoholic as a parent; yet ninety-five percent are left virtually ignored, fending for themselves in circumstances which many adults would consider personally intolerable.

Such children are powerless. While the alcoholic's spouse may seek counseling, commiserate with friends, or (worst case) file for divorce, the children can do nothing but "endure." Any outside figure who could intervene must get past Dad (or Mom) first.

Even worse, most children from alcoholic parents grow up not realizing their lives are abnormal: "This is the way life must be," the child senses.

Ironically the "sensing" does not continue; children in pain will adapt by numbing their feelings—or rather, by converting them into repressed anger, lowered self-esteem, destructive attention-getting; lack of trust; and loss of direction.

Our Secret Feelings will help therapists direct children to talk freely about their feelings. Creativity, games and fun are brought in to lighten any stress. Specific goals of the activities include:
- Gaining self-awareness;
- Accepting the disease of alcoholism;
- Being comfortable with one's feelings;
- Developing self-esteem in a troubled home;
- Facts about the disease of alcoholism;
- Learning about intimacy and friendship;
- Developing trust;
- Learning to enjoy childhood, despite pains;
- Discovering one is not alone.

Both the children and their group leader will discover new ways that interaction overcomes the withdrawal or anger which often afflicts COAs. The good habits of self expression can transform the child and nurture a dynamic adulthood.

Cat. # 207, ISBN 1-55691-020-7.................$9.95